Resilience Redefined

Thriving With Autoimmune Disease

written by Robyn Pineault &
Alissa Frazier | Denise Velarde | Mathew Embry |
Sara Stewart | Sarah St. John | Sarah Wilson

Copyright © 2023 ROBYN PINEAULT

All rights reserved. No part of this publication may be reproduced, distributed or transmitted in any form or by any means, including photocopying, recording, or other electronic or mechanical methods, without the prior written permission of the publisher, except in the case of brief quotations embodied in critical reviews and certain other non-commercial uses permitted by copyright law.

Resilience Redefined / Robyn Pineault
ISBN: 978-0-9951903-3-7

"It's your reaction to adversity, not adversity itself that determines how your life's story will develop."
– Dieter F. Uchtdorf

Contents

Foreword	8
From Multiple Sclerosis Patient To MS Coach	12
Athlete With A Purpose	33
MS Hope Founder & Advocate	56
Multiple Sclerosis Is My Sidekick	73
Strength In Faith	92
Trusting Your Intuition Through Illness	112
Healthier Because of Multiple Sclerosis	129

Foreword

"The oak fought the wind and was broken, the willow bent when it must and survived."
- Robert Jordan.

After publishing my first book in 2016, called Love Lost, Life Found, I had an itch to write another book. And to be honest, I toyed with the title Health Lost, Life Found. There are two distinct moments in my 40-some years where I've faced a challenge and had to discover how to live my life differently than I had previously. And technically, find it all over again. The first was when I called off a wedding, left a toxic relationship and then discovered a life that I truly love. Fast forward two and half years later, I was diagnosed with multiple sclerosis (MS) and had to discover how to create a life that I not only adore but one that I can thrive in. Although I was facing a health crisis, I knew I could find a life that I love again. However, the title wasn't fully resonating with me.

At the beginning of 2023, I felt called to create this book. But I didn't want to write this book on my own. Because strength is better in numbers and multiple stories of resilience are more powerful than one. And that's where Resilience Redefined was born.

In the pages of this book, you will follow along several transformative journeys through the lives of each author, who have faced the daunting challenge of living with autoimmune disease(s). "Resilience Redefined: Thriving with Autoimmune Disease" is a testament to the human spirit's unyielding capacity to triumph over adversity.

It is with great honor that I introduce you to my co-authors: Alissa Frazier, Denise Velarde, Mathew Embry, Sara Stewart, Sarah St. John, and Sarah Wilson – a collective of voices that are filled with resilience, hope, and determination. Each author brings a unique perspective, offering a flashlight that illuminates a path toward not just surviving but thriving with autoimmune disease.

The stories shared within this book cast a light on the struggles faced by millions around the globe, battling the unseen enemies within their own bodies. As you delve into each chapter, it becomes evident that each author is not simply recounting their battles with illness, but rather redefining their identities, reimagining their futures, and discovering newfound strength in the face of uncertainty.

The journey through these pages will be as diverse as the conditions they represent. From multiple sclerosis to Crohn's disease, each chapter covers unique challenges that autoimmune diseases present. Yet, through the tears, pain, and moments of despair, there lies an unwavering determination to rise above the limitations imposed by illness.

"Resilience Redefined" is not a prescription for a quick fix or a guide to eradicating autoimmune diseases altogether. Instead, it is an exploration of the human experience and the tenacity of the human spirit. We hope to remind you that true healing is not about restoring a perfect state of health but about embracing imperfections and embracing life with all its uncertainties.

Within these pages, you will find not only stories of struggle but also tales of transformation and triumph. The authors' collective wisdom woven together creates a resource of knowledge that extends beyond the boundaries of medical textbooks. We offer practical insights, emotional support, and the reassurance that you are not alone on this journey.

I urge you to read these stories with an open heart and an open mind. Allow the words to touch your soul and spark the embers of resilience within you. Let our courage inspire you to redefine your own narrative, to find strength in vulnerability, and to embrace the beauty of resilience building.

In closing, I extend my deepest gratitude to the other six remarkable authors who poured their hearts and souls into these pages. Your willingness to share your vulnerabilities and victories has created inspiration that will undoubtedly touch the lives of countless readers.

With utmost admiration,

Robyn Pineault
Multiple Sclerosis Thriver

"Resilience is not about avoiding the challenges and struggles of life; it's about facing them head-on with courage and perseverance."
- Unknown

1

From Multiple Sclerosis Patient To MS Coach

Alissa Frazier

Resilience means not giving up or losing sight of hope. We all have our "bad" or "down" days, but how we come back from them is what counts. There is always hope.

I'd like to dedicate my chapter to my husband Scott and my parents. Scott, each day I am floored by your support and unwavering love. Thank you for always being my rock and on my side. Mom and Dad, thank you for teaching me to question everything. If I didn't, the story in this chapter wouldn't have been possible.

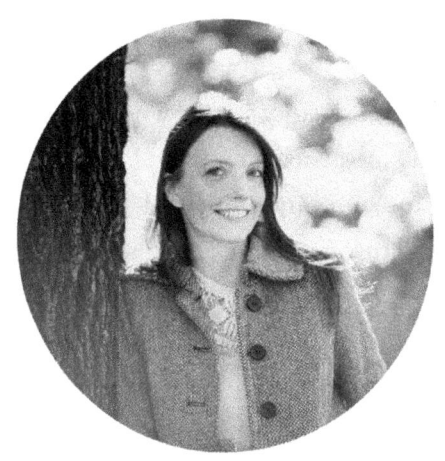

ALISSA FRAZIER

Alissa is the practitioner and blogger behind LissMS. She is a Licensed Mental Health Counselor, Certified Personal Trainer, Nutritional Therapy Practitioner and AIP Certified Coach. Alissa works remotely with individuals who have Multiple Sclerosis and other autoimmune diseases to help them create a lifestyle that helps them to feel better in their bodies. She utilizes a 3-pronged approach including diet, movement and stress management changes to help individuals improve their symptoms, feel better in their skin and create a lifestyle that improves their health. Alissa is based near Boston, MA and lives with her husband and 3 cats. She loves being outdoors and can usually be found hiking or lifting weights.

Diagnosis Story

My diagnosis story started when I was very young. You see when I look back on my life, I can see how various risk factors for autoimmunity and multiple sclerosis were present all throughout my childhood and adolescence.

I had repeated ear infections as a child, which meant multiple rounds of antibiotics. I was born in May, which brings with it a 20% higher risk of developing MS[1]. I lived in places at higher latitudes that didn't have year-round sun, which meant less vitamin D production in my body. I got mono in ninth grade[2], then kept getting mystery infection after mystery infection throughout the rest of high school.

And the most interesting part of my pre-diagnosis life is that I used to describe feeling as though my body was attacking itself. The only record I have of getting diagnosed is a Facebook post, where I lament my past self by saying "One must not joke about their body attacking

---

[1] https://www.nationalmssociety.org/About-the-Society/News/Month-of-Birth-May-Influence-Risk-of-MS-by-Promoti
[2] https://www.nature.com/articles/s41579-022-00770-5

themselves." Some part of me must've known what was coming even way back then.

But first, let's rewind to about three months before I wrote that Facebook post. I had just turned 24; I was in graduate school for mental health counseling and working at Target when not in school. Unfortunately, I was also about a year into an abusive relationship.

To say my life was busy is an understatement.

I remember one afternoon while working at Target, I was walking down the main aisle and I noticed that my vision was a little blurry. It wasn't 100% blurry like if you got your eyes dilated at the eye doctor. It was blotchier, like if you were wearing glasses and there were a few water droplets on them. I could still see; it was just weird.

Then not long after, I noticed I had a weird electrical feeling when I tilted my head down. The year before, I had back surgery, so I just thought those two were related. I made an appointment with my neurosurgeon for later that month and didn't think anything else of it.

Eventually, I got fed up with my vision and made an appointment with an eye doctor. The eye doctor said the exam looked fine and I had 20/20 vision, but I needed to go get an MRI immediately.

"Immediately, eh?"

That seemed a little bit dramatic, but OK, off I went.

I got a call from the eye doctor a few days later with the MRI results. He said I didn't have a brain tumor (which I didn't even know was a possibility) but I should go see a neurologist immediately.

Again, I thought that was dramatic, but I found a neurologist and made an appointment.

He listened to my symptoms and ordered more tests, including MRIs, blood tests, visual field tests, and a spinal tap.

The whole process to get all these tests completed took about three months, which I've heard is fast for an MS diagnosis. I've heard many other stories from people who were struggling with symptoms for 5–10 years before a doctor was able to give a definitive diagnosis.

When I finally sat down with the neurologist at the end of August to get the results from everything, he told me that he was confident I had MS.

Because of his findings, he suggested I go on medication right away to help prevent any other relapses or progression. He handed me a giant stack of drug company pamphlets about their latest and greatest medication, told me to pick one, and sent me on my way.

Now, I had heard about MS before, but I had no idea what it really meant until I went home and googled it. To say I was shocked by what I read was an understatement. I didn't quite understand how I, being a relatively healthy 24-year-old, could wind up with such a debilitating disease so quickly.

I figured I should listen to the doctor, so I chose a medication from the stack and carried on with my life. Remember, I was still in an abusive relationship and in grad school at this time, so being diagnosed with MS fell low on my list of priorities; after all, besides a little eye blurriness and an odd feeling in my back, I felt "fine."

Over the next few years, I graduated from grad school, got a new job, kicked the crappy boyfriend to the curb, and got a much better boyfriend. Things were looking good.

In fact, things were going so well I started a new hobby: running. I did a bunch of races, including a few half marathons. Inevitably, I would always get giant blisters when I did that distance. At one point, one of those blisters got infected. In order to help heal that infection, I had to stop taking my MS medication for a little while.

If I didn't mention it before, I was, and still am, rather stubborn.

This stubbornness coupled with considerable unprocessed anger about my MS diagnosis led me to continue without the medication even after I cleared the infection. The medication I had picked had the fewest side effects but was also the one that you had to inject into your body every day. Daily injections got old to me quickly, as I'm sure you can imagine.

Eventually, the new, much better boyfriend (who is now my husband) convinced me to go back on the medication. However, I believe the eventual damage was already done.

Deciding to Take Care of Myself

Fast forward a few months to a nice Saturday in early June. I woke up, ready to go to work, when I realized I was unable to feel the entire right side of my body—from my arm, across my back, and all the way down to my leg. I immediately called my neurologist's office, talked to the neurologist on call, and got in for an MRI. A few days later, I had my first steroid infusion and my first official relapse.

Unfortunately, my time away from medication started a series of relapses. I had three relapses within about a year and a half, which is kind of fast in the MS world. I had symptoms like numbness, tingling, pain, exhaustion, burning, and cognitive issues.

At my breaking point, I remember standing in the conference room at work, waiting for my coffee to brew. I didn't realize that I had tears streaming down my face until my boss, who thankfully was also a good friend, came in and asked what was wrong.

I was in so much pain and was so exhausted, I knew something needed to change.

At some point before this moment, I had gone down several internet research rabbit holes. During one of those sessions, I found information on the Autoimmune Protocol, a diet designed for individuals with autoimmune diseases to lessen their inflammation and find out which foods are most helpful and which ones are not helpful for them.

The idea that food could be this helpful was revolutionary to me. I was shocked to learn that what we eat has that much of an impact on our bodies. It seems kind of like common sense now, but it was groundbreaking and life-changing for me at the time.

Starting the Autoimmune Protocol is no easy task. I have now come to call it "Paleo on steroids." There are quite a few foods that you eliminate during the initial elimination phase. This is exactly what stopped me from trying it when I first read about it, but my symptoms had been much less severe back then and I hadn't felt like it was worth the effort.

Finally, in January 2015, 6 years after my initial diagnosis, I waved the white flag and started the Autoimmune Protocol.

To say my results were life-changing would be an understatement. Within four months, the pain, sensory symptoms, and complete exhaustion were all pretty much resolved.

This experience opened a whole new world for me of holistic and alternative medicine. I began to look at everything in my life through this lens. I realized there was so much more I could be doing for myself, my health, and my disease progression. I knew I didn't want to leave it up to only medication anymore. I couldn't; my life depended on it.

This led me to do a ton more research and basically overhaul my entire life over the next few years. I changed how I worked out, moving from only cardio and running to more of a strength-based exercise paradigm. I added supplements to shore up some nutritional deficiencies and help my body to function better. I also got honest about the significant role that stress was playing in my life. This led to the biggest change of all: quitting my job.

There's a saying that goes something like, "You can't heal in the same environment where you got sick." I don't think I really knew this yet, but I did everything I could to change my environment.

And it helped.

The Tools I Use to Thrive

I was so encouraged by my own transformation; that I knew I needed to tell others about this possibility for themselves. On top of having my mental health counselling license, I became a Nutritional Therapy Practitioner, a Certified Personal Trainer, and eventually an Autoimmune Protocol Coach.

I started helping others walk through this process of changing their diet, their exercise, their relationship to stress, and basically their entire lives.

Although everyone is a little bit different and needs different things for their bodies, my starting points for clients are usually very similar. I'd love to share them with you as well.

Addition Before Subtraction

When I first meet with clients, they often have an expectation that I'm about to blow up their food world—that I'm going to require so many things to be eliminated they won't know what they can eat. However, I start in a much different place. We work on what to add to their diet before we take anything away.

I didn't start like this, but I sure wish I did. As I mentioned above, I jumped in and started with eliminations first. If I could go back in time, I'd do it this way instead.

I would have started here:
- Adding more fruits and vegetables, especially dark leafy greens and brightly colored berries and veggies (the deeper the color, the more nutrients)
- Swapping unhealthy fats (canola oil, fried foods) for healthy fats (nuts, seeds, avocado, coconut)
- Adding more seafood and shellfish to recipe rotations

These small changes alone could have made a big impact on the amount of nutrients I was getting in a day.

Mindful Eating

Our lives are incredibly busy. Between work, household chores, kids' activities, pets, and events, we're always on the go. One of the things that suffers when we are so busy is mealtimes. Many of my clients come to me with habits of eating on the go, in the car, or only have a few minutes to get in a meal before they're off to the next thing they must do.

When we eat like this, most of the time we are eating when our nervous system is in a sympathetic state. This means we are eating in fight or flight, which is not optimal.

Many of us are functioning in this state more than we think. When we are experiencing or feeling stress, most likely we are in a state of fight or flight. One of the things that happens in this state is that digestion shuts off because if we really did need to fight or fight, we don't need to be digesting food at the same time.

This means that when we eat in a hurried or stressed state, our body is not fully digesting the food we're eating. This can lead to digestive complications like bloating, gas, and even dysbiosis (where "bad" bacteria outnumber the "good" and further create issues).

I'm not sharing this to shame anyone. We've all eaten like this, including myself. Sometimes it's a necessity, depending on the situation.

But if this is a common habit, and you are dealing with some level of G.I. distress, mindful eating might be something to try. Here are some tips:

- Before you eat, sit down and take at least five deep breaths. Pray or meditate for a minute on the food you're about to eat. Feel gratitude and appreciation.
- During meals, be mindful of what you're eating and chew your food for approximately 30 chews. (The more liquid the food is in your mouth, the easier it will be for your body to digest.)
- Put your fork down between bites if needed.

Even if we can't do this all the time, that's okay. Just try at least once a day to start.

Hydrate

Another area that is an opportunity for most people is hydration. I know it sounds like something that is simple, but most of us are not getting enough water each day.

Being optimally hydrated helps with so many things. It helps our digestion to function better, our joints to work better, and our cells to communicate better… I could go on.

An easy-to-calculate guideline, which I'm sure you've heard by now, is to take your body weight in pounds, divide that in half, and that's your target ounces of water a day. This is a good starting place with water intake.

Different situations might call for more i.e., higher temperatures or exercise, so keep that in mind as well.

I'm all about small steps as you can tell, so if you find that you are far away from that number, just add another glass a day and start there.

A few other things that help myself and my clients get enough water is using a cool water bottle that you enjoy or trying one of the water tracking apps that exist.

Movement > Exercise

Many people have negative preconceived notions and ideas about "exercise." It makes sense, especially when society has such strong messages about exercise, like "no pain, no gain." But that approach usually doesn't work for those of us diagnosed with an autoimmune disease or chronic illness. It certainly didn't work for me when I was trying to reintegrate movement into my life after my relapses.

When I was struggling to exercise again after my relapses, I had an epiphany. I had been thinking of exercise like I used to, that I needed to have an intense workout for it to "count." But then I realized that my body was different, so I had to approach exercise differently.

Instead of thinking only about exercise, I opened to the idea of swapping the word (and idea) of exercise for movement. I found that using the word "movement" wasn't as constrictive as "exercise" was and didn't have as many stereotypical parameters set around it.

To illustrate my point, if I told you, "Make sure you get 30 minutes of exercise a day" or "Make sure you get 30 minutes of movement a day," which feels more doable? I bet you'd say movement.

Is gardening exercise? Maybe, but it sure is movement.
Is playing with your kids' exercise? Maybe, but it sure is movement.

See where I'm going with this?

Our bodies were designed to be moving, so adding a little bit wherever feels comfortable would be great.

Maybe you work in the garden for 20 minutes, hula hoop with your kids, or go for a slow walk with your dog. Whatever you do, make sure you do it because you want to, not because it's something society expects of you.

Awareness

I saved my most important point for last.

Up until a few years ago, I was living my life on autopilot, unaware of myself. I didn't realize how much this affected my life and my perceptions.

Living on autopilot is exactly what it sounds like: moving through the world doing the same things, reacting the same way, thinking the same things, etc. Which makes sense, our brain naturally likes to conserve energy - which means doing the same thing every day. But is that most helpful? Sometimes not.

To add a layer to this, most of us aren't living in a zen autopilot mode where we're super calm and chill all the time. We're in a "rushing around then crashing" autopilot mode. This often means our nervous system is dysregulated, and we're bouncing from fight/flight (rushing around) to freeze (crash).

Most of my clients come to me living on autopilot mode and with dysregulated nervous systems too. There are many reasons for this autopilot and nervous system dysfunction that we try to function in, much too many for me to get into right now, but this is how I started to be aware and move out of autopilot.

I created a few times in the day, ideally two or three, to check in with myself. I just stopped whatever I was doing, took a few deep breaths, and asked myself: *What are you thinking, feeling, and doing?* I didn't try to change it at first. I just wanted to bring awareness to what is affecting me throughout the day.

Then I asked myself, *Do I need anything at this moment?* Then I worked to give myself what I needed.

In my opinion, the best way to remember to do this is not to remember—meaning, you should set an alarm or reminder in the morning, sometime midday, and in the evening. Ideally, it will pop up on your phone (the one time I'm in favor of notifications) so you can see it easily.

Here's an example of this in action:

Your check-in alarm goes off at 10:30 in the morning. You just got home from running a few errands and you are thinking of what you must do this evening to prep for dinner. You're feeling really tired, and you already need a break, but you were about to just do the next thing on your to-do list because you "should." Instead, when you stop to check in you realize just how tired you are, and you decide to go sit down for a little bit and take a rest.

This doesn't seem like much of anything, and in terms of "doing" you're not "doing" much. But you really are. In these little moments of awareness, you are starting to break out of autopilot mode. You are starting to become more connected to yourself and your needs.

We can't really change anything that we are not aware of, so in my world, awareness is the first step and the most important one.

Mindset Work

In all the work I've done and the changes I've made, the most profound has come from my mindset and stress management work. For me, this really means nervous system work.

Remember when I talked about finding the Autoimmune Protocol? Through that, I also found a community of people who were working on helping themselves in various ways. This was groundbreaking for me: up until that point, I had been angry and had a view of "why me" and "this isn't fair" about getting an MS diagnosis.

For the first time, I was around people who didn't think that way. I'm not saying they loved having an autoimmune disease or thought it was fair—I would imagine if they had the choice, they wouldn't have MS or the autoimmune disease they were dealing with—but instead of thinking, *"why me?"* they thought, *"what is this showing me or teaching me?"*

In my case, I realized that MS was giving me an opportunity to care for myself in a much deeper and more loving way. Because up until my diagnosis, I hadn't been doing the best I could for myself. Through this mindset shift, I was able to process my anger and move toward acceptance. This didn't mean I was suddenly happy about having MS; for me it was more that I acknowledged that yes, I have MS, and that means I need to support myself.

I realized I had been living on autopilot and with a dysregulated nervous system for a long time. From early adolescence, I had been stuck going back and forth between depression (freeze) and anxiety (fight/flight). When I started to become aware of my thoughts, emotions, and actions, I realized how the autopilot pattern I had been living in wasn't very helpful to my future health. It's been one of the hardest parts of myself to work on, but also the most helpful.

Resilience Redefined

In the first few months of my diet changes, someone close to me said, "I respect you for what you're doing for yourself, but it's too late for me."

This broke my heart to hear because, in my opinion, it's never too late. It's never too late to try to improve your health in any way. Ps. 10 years later, this person I mentioned above did make a lot of positive changes in their life. Proving you're never too old, but there absolutely is a right time.

There are a million reasons why change is hard. Some days it will feel easy, some days it will feel downright impossible. But that's okay. It's okay to have setbacks now and again; we all do. It's okay to have to start over sometimes; we all do.

Healing is not a linear process, as much as we'd like to make it that way. There will be ups and downs, days where you feel like a rock star and some, where you want to hide under a rock. It's all okay and it's all part of the process.

The only thing we CAN'T do is give up...

2

Athlete With A Purpose

Denise Velarde

Resilience is my superpower of adapting to all variations in life. It is how I conquer any and all hurdles that come my way at any given time.

To my sweet mother, Carmen
Who is the greatest example of what it means to live
fearlessly.

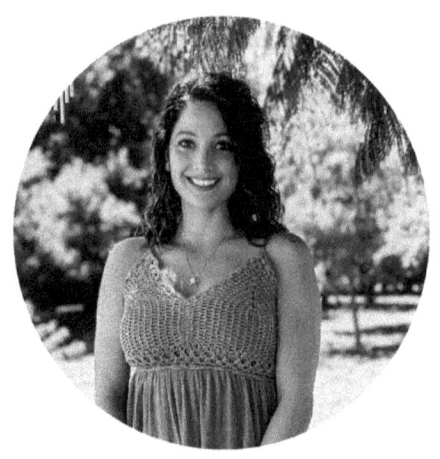

DENISE VELARDE

Denise Velarde is a health enthusiast who played various sports growing up and had an interest in exercise and diet at an early age. In college, she studied and earned degrees in health science, social and behavioral sciences, and psychology. After being diagnosed with multiple sclerosis (MS) in 2015 and having an unsuccessful recovery with disease-modifying drugs (DMDs), she decided to use her knowledge and skills in how to heal using a holistic approach. She wanted to do more than just share her journey publicly to inspire others to live well with MS and has recently become an ambassador for the Overcoming MS community. She aspires and is passionate to help others navigate life while dealing with this disease. In her free time, you can find her at the finish line of a trail race, at the gym, or camping in the great outdoors.

Diagnosis Story

I was sitting in the passenger seat of our car in my gym clothes, annoyed by the traffic on the highway and accompanied by the worst headache I'd ever experienced. I kept telling myself that the headache would go away after exercising. But after an hour of sitting in traffic, it was worse, and my vision seemed a bit blurred. It was hard to keep my eyes open. "Drop me off at home. I have a migraine and need to rest." He kept one hand on the steering wheel and grabbed my hand with the other.

"I'll drop you off at home. Take a bath, relax. I will come back with your favorite food."

The bathroom was steamy and smelled like eucalyptus. As I began to scrub my body, I realized my left leg was asleep. *Ugh, dumb traffic*, I thought. *I was sitting in the same position for too long; I can't believe it caused my leg to fall asleep.* Scrubbing continued and I realized the right side of my abdomen was also numb. I got out and began to pat myself all over my body, panicking... my entire right side, front and back, was numb. *Okay, Dee, it's asleep, that's all.* Relax. I walked upstairs to change into my pyjamas, my gut telling me something was wrong. I stopped as soon as I made it to the room; I had a thought. *When I was a kid, I stomped my foot to wake it up. Brilliant! Let me wake it up.* I skipped the getting dressed part and began to run up and down the stairs.

"I thought you wanted to skip the gym and not work out but here you are, doing... some form of exercise." He laughed in confusion, holding the bag that read Wokcano.

"Oh, sushi! Yum! Okay, I'm coming." I put my clothes on and ran down the stairs to the living room. We sat on the couch, getting ready to watch our show while we ate. "I wasn't running to work out," I explained. "My leg is asleep. Well, my entire right side, front and back, from head to toe. It's never been asleep this long. But it's okay, I'm sure it'll wake up soon. Let's eat. Hit play!"

He stopped my hand from grabbing the remote. "What is going on? Are you okay? Here, take this Tylenol for your headache."

"Yes, I'm fine. Do you know that feeling when your foot is asleep? Feels like springs when you walk or stomp. It's okay, it'll go away, I'm sure." I grabbed the remote and we watched our show. I don't recall anything else from that night. I don't know what happened in the episode nor do I remember the sushi rolls I ate.

At 7 am the next day I stood in front of the mirror. I smiled, lifted my arm up, stuck my tongue out. *Okay. It's not that. But I need to go to the ER.* I ran to my closet, grabbed my medical card from my purse, and called the emergency number provided on the back. The nurse answered in a high happy pitch. "Hi! My name is Melina, is this an emergency?"

I could hear her smile on the other end. "Hello, I am okay, no open wounds, but this is an emergency. I am completely numb on the right side of my body. Front and back from head to toe. It's now been 12 to 14 hours…" I continued to explain in detail. She then asked me a series of questions that led me to realize that I had been experiencing horrible headaches for the last two weeks—migraines with a sharp sudden pain in the right temple causing double blurred vision. It would remain blurry for quite some time and carry on to the next day on and off. She told me that based on the answers I provided, all seemed to be normal things we experience. Icing my leg for 30 minutes four times a day should help.

I quickly dialed one of my sisters. "Heeey sissy, what's up?" she answered. I could tell by the sound of her voice that she had just woken up not too long ago and was walking around her house, so I didn't feel too bad for calling her so early.

"Hey, so don't freak out," I said. I heard her take a deep breath, about to say something. "I'm fine," I said quickly, then gave her the 411. I told her Mousa was taking me to the ER over at Henry Mayo down the street from our house. "Please don't tell Mom or anyone else. I don't want anyone to worry. Especially Mom. Not until I know what is going on. I just want to tell someone where I will be in case, in case… it is something bad."

"Got it, okay, I agree. But Dee, make sure to keep me updated on everything. I'll talk to you soon."

"Wait! Bren!"

"Yes?" she said, catching my voice before hanging up.

"If anything, I'll have Mousa keep you updated. I most likely won't have my phone on me if they run tests, etc."

"Okay, I'll text him now to let him know I'll be expecting updates. Love you, sissy."

"Love you too, Bren."

I walked into the ER and headed toward the receptionist. There was a lady in front of me with her child. As I stood there waiting for my turn, all I could think was that this was not where I wanted to be on a Saturday morning. I began to look around. It was busy, loud, and chaotic.

"I can help you here," the receptionist said. I looked at her, and my mouth opened, but no words came out. Mousa gave her my name and pulled me close to his side. I snapped out of it, answered her questions, and explained why I was there.

"You definitely need to see someone. I will need your ID and insurance card to check you in."

I handed it over to her. "Thank you."

After an hour the doctor finally came in to talk to me. He ordered bloodwork and a CT scan. It was the first time in my life getting a CT done. It was weird; I began to feel uncertain, and worried. I don't recall finishing the test or walking back to the gurney. The next thing I knew, I was waking up to the voice of my doctor. "Cat scan and bloodwork look good. Nothing is wrong; it's probably just stress." He struggled to get his hands into the pockets of his white coat. "I'll send you home with...."

"Excuse me, but I am not going home," I interrupted. My voice was trembling yet stern, my eyes hard on his. "Something is terribly wrong. I know it! You are an ER doctor who is under constant stress, do you ever get numb like this? Please, I am not going home."

He stared at me for a minute; I couldn't help but notice the bags under his eyes, his pale face that could use some sun. In a hopeless voice, he said, "Fine, the only other test I can think of at this point is an MRI."

"That's fine with me! Where do I go?" You'd think I would remember my first MRI. But like so many other things, I didn't. After the test I was lying in the hospital bed, fighting to keep my eyes open. I was cold, but at least the bed was filled with a few squishy pillows that made it comforting for me. I turned my body to face Mousa. I could see it all over his face. He was sad, worried, tired, trying to hide it and stay strong for me. He caught me looking at him then looked past me. From my peripheral vision, I saw the doctor making his way into the room.

He took a deep breath. "So, I'm glad we did the MRI, there are some..." It all went silent from there.

Everything stopped, frozen in time.

"Call Bren," I said. I put my head to my knees. *Please God, please! Don't let it be cancer. I'm not mad at you. I promise I'm not. Whatever it is... I will fight, I won't give up, I won't be afraid, I won't lose faith. Just please don't let it be cancer.*

I awoke in another room; I had been admitted. My sister Bren was by my bedside. "Mom is on her way. How are you feeling?"

"Fine, I suppose, but I'm not sure what is going on. The doctor said we need to run tests to find out."

"Dee, you have a diagnosis. I was informed when I got the call. Don't you know what it is? You already did tests; the MRI shows you have multiple sclerosis. But they need to confirm it with a spinal tap and a few more tests." Her eyes searched mine with a sad yet more concerned look, wondering why I was not aware of this.

"Oh," I said. "I don't recall much. All I know is that I was downstairs, the doctor entered the room, and now I'm awake and you are here..." I shrugged a shoulder and thought to myself, What on God's green earth is multiple sclerosis?

My time in the hospital is a bit of a distant memory for me. I recall my body taking up space there. I recall not being able to sit on the toilet because the cold seat caused "pain" to the right buttock (my sister customized the seat by wrapping a towel on the right side of it). Anything cold such as water, objects, and even slightly cold hands caused pain and made me feel as if my entire body was going to power down like a robot. It felt as if every ounce of my energy was being sucked out of me and my entire world was about to be erased. It was hard for me to read without skipping lines, I was confusing some letters or forgot what some of them were, and I had no energy or strength to walk. After two weeks of being in the hospital, I was happy to hear that I could go home.

Deciding to Take Care of Myself

I was sent off with a new medication, Copaxone. This was an injection that I had to give myself three times a week. It was painful, it did not improve my symptoms, I was continually getting sick, and it made me sick. I took this medication for two to three years. The third year was interrupted by my medical insurance being terminated because I was starting a new job and my new insurance would not begin until 90 days after hire. During that time, I feared my MS would get worse. I couldn't afford the medication. A month's supply cost $7,300, which is almost $88,000 a year. Stress was now taking over, which caused me to be more stressed out. And many of us who have MS (or any autoimmune disease) know stress can cause flares—or worse. Little did I know this situation was a blessing in disguise.

I began to do some research of my own. I was eager to find answers on how to manage my MS without medication and if that was even possible. After hours of being on the internet and feeling overwhelmed, I shut it off and let the tears come down. I turned up the music in my room so no one would hear me cry. It was one of those ugly cries. You know, where you put your face in the pillow because it's a loud cry with weird sounds coming out? Yeah, that kind of cry.

Maybe it was the position my body was in, similar to when I put my head to my knees that day in the ER, but I suddenly remembered that I had told myself I would fight, not give up, be afraid, or lose faith. And just like that, I picked my head up from the pillow. I wiped my tears, took a deep breath, drank some water, and walked to my closet mirror. I stood there for maybe eight minutes. As I stared at myself, I noticed two things: I was filled with worry, and I felt hope that overrode the worry. Without taking my eyes off my reflection, I took two steps back and said a verse that came to my mind that very moment.

"SHE IS CLOTHED IN STRENGTH AND DIGNITY AND SHE LAUGHS WITHOUT FEAR OF THE FUTURE."

That night I did not sleep as I searched the web for answers. Then I found it: a YouTube video of Terry Wahls, a doctor with MS who had been on the same medication as I was, who had not been getting any better just as I wasn't. A doctor who found the answers on how to heal with food. I ordered her book that same night. Thanks to Amazon Prime, I received the book two days later. I could not stop reading and that very same day, I went cold turkey and eliminated foods that are known to make MS worse. Months later, I could feel the difference within. I had energy again, my symptoms were gone, and I felt great. I could not stop reading medical journals or listening to any and all MS-related podcasts. I discovered research scientist, Ashton Embry, professor and founder of neuroepidemiology, George Jelinek, and professor of neurology, Roy Swank. All of them not only believe in diet and exercise to conquer MS but have the supporting data to show for it.

Nine months later, I showed up for my follow-up with my neurologist. I was sitting on the patient bed as he reviewed the MRI that I had done the week prior to our visit. "Miss Denise, your newest MRI looks beautiful. There are no new lesions, no active lesions. In fact, the previous lesions seem to be smaller, which is great news and means that the medication is working. I will put in a prescription for a refill..."

My chuckle stopped whatever he was going to say next. He stared at me with a smirk on his face. I hopped down from the bed with a smile on my face. "No, doctor, I don't need a refill; I have not been on medication for nine months now."

His entire demeanor changed; he was dismayed. "Excuse me?"

"That's right! I didn't have insurance coverage for that long."

"Well." He cleared his throat. "What have you been doing?" he asked with a nervous laugh.

"I cranked up my exercise regimen and cut out gluten, sugar, and dairy. Nothing but nature's best foods," I said, smiling ear to ear, and began to list it all. "A variety of veggies, fruits, seeds, nuts, fermented things I never knew existed, seafood, chicken here and there, and plenty of journaling."

"It seems to have done its job, but it's time to go back on medication." It was my turn to stand there confused and I thought to myself, *What the French toast? Did he just dismiss the fact that I'm doing great?* I snapped out of it as he said, "Okay, we will follow up in three months, your prescription will be ready for pickup by tomorrow."

"I'm not picking it up. I am doing great and even forget that I have MS most days. I am no longer feeling sick or getting reactions from the injections, I have no flare-ups, and most importantly I have my MRI to show for it." He told me it would be malpractice if he did not give me medication. But I stood my ground. We came to an agreement that I would continue to use food and exercise as medicine. At any point, if I felt changes that needed medical attention, I would not hesitate to reach out and start medication.

A year had gone by since I saw my neurologist. Everything was fine until I added a lot to my plate. I started school and working full time. I had no life. I was getting 4–5 hours of sleep and was stressed out trying to keep up with studying, homework, and my relationship. I barely ate most days because I chose sleep over eating. Whenever I did eat—which was more like snacking because I was always on the run—I ate packaged foods such as "healthy" chips, protein bars, and bread that wasn't gluten or dairy free. Here and there I also had some mixed drinks or wine. Even though I tried to justify that it was only a little bit, that little bit added up to a lot. The perfect recipe for a relapse.

It was my first relapse in five years since I was diagnosed. It was worse than my diagnosis, to be honest. I was lethargic, it hurt to walk, my leg muscles felt weak, and my face and eye sockets had this sharp pain I'd never felt. My torso along with my left arm was numb and both my legs felt as if they were on fire. The brain fog I experienced scared me the most. I was very forgetful and forgot a lot of things even just a couple of minutes after they happened. I could not think clearly enough to continue my thought processes. It was as if my brain would shut off and that was that. I remember sitting on the chair with the steroid IV thinking, *This is all my fault. If I hadn't put the crap I ate and drank into my body, I wouldn't be here.*

On the last day of my steroid infusion, I met with another neurologist. I no longer had relapsing-remitting MS (RRMS) but secondary progressive MS (SPMS), according to my doctor, and he determined it was best he transferred my care to someone who had more experience. Hearing this devastated me because I was the one to blame. He explained that because I was now SPMS, I would need second-tier medication: infusions. He named three for me to read about prior to meeting with my new doctor. Let me tell you, none of these infusions were appealing to me. I not only read about them but searched medical journals and trials about each one and was not sold on any.

My interaction with the new neurologist made me sick to my stomach. She was not empathetic at all. She stormed into the room, told me her name, and immediately started stating the new lesions in my brain and spinal cord. I began to cry, apologized, and told her I needed a moment. She stayed silent for a few seconds then said, "You are young. You don't want to end up in a wheelchair in a year now do you?" When she said this, something inside of me snapped. I felt my blood boiling. I looked right at her and began to breathe heavily. She then said, "I think you are having a panic attack. This is normal, especially after being on steroids. But just take a deep breath and hear me out. You need to go on rituximab..."

I stood up and laughed a little bit in disbelief that this was happening. Are you kidding me? You see I'm not okay and you are continuing this conversation as if nothing is happening? I walked out.

I gave myself a pep talk out loud when I got home. "I have done this before. I have the MRI to prove that with diet, exercise, sleep, and journaling I can heal and thrive. I will do it again but better. I won't let my guard down." I gave myself about two weeks to calm down and put myself back together. Then I made an appointment with a different neurologist. She was supportive of my decision, but this healing process was a difficult one.

I went from lifting dumbbells 30 pounds or more to struggling to lift a 5-pound dumbbell. From doing 225-pound leg presses to no weight on the leg press machine. The change happened from one day to the next—literally overnight. I felt weak. Walking from my bedroom to the kitchen wore me out, the double vision was back, and I had electric shocks running up and down my spine. I had a hard time running due to vertigo-like symptoms. The strangest two symptoms of all were that my depth perception was off and that whenever metal such as a razor blade touched my body, I felt intense zaps. I had to dig deep within myself because I refused to give up. I refused to let this disease win. I refused to let it cause fear and stop me from what I know I am capable of. I said it out loud again.

"SHE IS CLOTHED IN STRENGTH AND DIGNITY AND SHE LAUGHS WITHOUT FEAR OF THE FUTURE."

The Tools I Use to Thrive

I read various medical journals that focused on the correlation of diet and exercise with MS, as well as medication with MS so that I can reassure myself on the decision I was making. I began to eat whole foods again and made sure I got plenty of rest every night. I learned how to incorporate strategies to reduce stress, educated myself on minerals and vitamins that I can ingest directly from foods, and I began to cook more at home. I also learned of the importance of gut health and therefore began to include fermented foods, fiber, and probiotics in my diet.

I made it a point to talk to others who also have MS (or any other autoimmune disease) so that we can learn from one another and so that I can help others in any way I can. I re-evaluated my circle which was very important because some did not truly understand what I am up against. They would make ignorant comments which had an impact on me emotionally because it made me feel alone, misunderstood, and as if I had no support. But I knew that the only important factor here was healing my body. I believed in myself and knew changes were happening. I felt it and within time it showed.

Clean Eating

Deciding to eat a certain way was an easy job because it is one thing, I know I have complete control over.

However, I am not always perfect with it, but I don't let it bring me down - re-focus and move along. Knowing that whole foods have healed me before has led me to my ultimate decision to continue to avoid processed/packaged "foods". I eat a variety of fish and some chicken for my protein intake. Plenty of vegetables and fruits - especially the dark leafy green and brightly colored ones, raw honey (which helps with my sweet tooth), herbal teas, cod liver oil, flaxseed oil, raw nuts, nut butter, and seeds for healthy fats. I also avoid foods I am sensitive to in order to avoid inflammation and a leaky gut.

Exercise

As time went by, I could feel my body healing. I continued to work out *every single day* regardless of the tingles and numbness because I could feel the symptoms subsiding. Again, comments would arise, "You are overworking your body, for someone with MS, maybe you need to not work out so much." BLAH BLAH BLAH was all I heard. I let that be background noise and paid no attention. I'm sure they meant well. However, I am glad I did not stop; I became in tune with my body where I could easily recognize when to push harder, or if I needed recovery time or more. Listening to my body is key. On days I feel I need to rest; I do yoga or take the dogs for a walk instead of a vigorous workout. All movement counts! Stretching, and massaging my body as much as I work out is also very important for my healing as well.

Mindset Work

It is important for me to have "me time". This is the time when I can pay attention to my thoughts and have a clear understanding of how I am dealing with everything around me. I let my mind wander and I acknowledge each thought carefully as they come. Doing this helps me get an understanding of how those thoughts influence me emotionally. This is important because, in turn, those feelings impact my acts of service towards myself, my family and my friends. Another strategy I use for mindset work is practicing mindfulness. It not only reduces my stress levels, but it allows me to slow down, connect with nature, and embrace the little things. It is so easy to do and rewarding at the same time because it fills me with gratitude.

Little did I know that using the above tools to thrive is just the beginning of a new me. My symptoms have gone away. I ran my longest trail race to date at 20.7 miles—and shortly after, I completed a 132-mile Ragnar relay race with a group of MS warriors. How awesome is it that we were the first team composed solely of people with MS to ever run a Ragnar race? We ran from sunup to sundown facing temperatures that changed from super cold in the morning to dry heat during the day. Months later I signed up for a bodybuilding competition, where I placed second in my division. I am currently training for my first ultra-trail race which is to take place in December 2023. This is more than just goals. It's my way of knowing that I am okay because my body is capable of physical achievements and my mental health is constantly adapting and getting stronger. This lifestyle is my medication.

Now, if you are wondering if the unwelcome comments ever stopped, they didn't. I do wonder when someone will ask me how I am doing with my MS because believe it or not, it's rare when someone does. I'd like to believe that the reason they don't ask is because they forgot I have MS since I am doing so great. I hope I can inspire others to live a healthy lifestyle. This journey is not easy, it has no end, and it is indeed a beautiful disaster. It has taught me how to be resilient, embrace being vulnerable and adapt to any battles life throws my way in order to rise above MS.

We all have strength within. We just need to find it,

hold on tight to it, never lose hope, and most importantly, laugh without fear of the future!

3

MS Hope Founder & Advocate

Mathew Embry

For me, resilience is a dedication to well-being, reinforced by a commitment to no cheat days, understanding that each day and every decision significantly enhances our ability to self-improve. Consistent, mindful choices are integral to fostering optimal health, equipping us with the strength to overcome adversity and thrive amidst life's challenges.

I dedicate this chapter to the memory of my mother, Joan Embry, who courageously sailed into a storm to save me and many others worldwide.

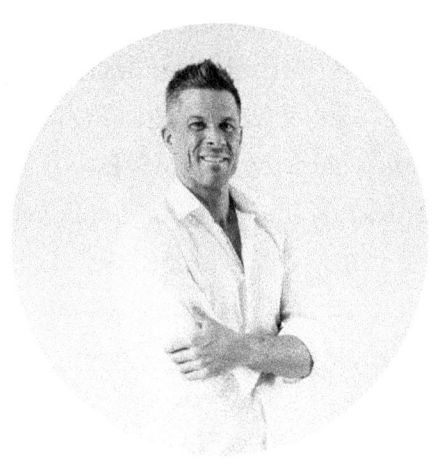

MATHEW EMBRY

Mathew Embry is an internationally recognized filmmaker, an MS advocate, and the President and Founder of MS Hope (www.mshope.com). Diagnosed with MS in 1995, he redefined his life around the principles of resilience and conscious daily choices, demonstrating that living with MS is not an endpoint, but a beginning of a health-focused journey. Today, he is symptom-free, thanks to the science-based strategies found on mshope.com.

As the son of the founders of Direct-MS, Dr. Ashton Embry and Joan Embry, Mathew's advocacy roots run deep. He continued his parents' work by producing and directing the influential documentary Living Proof, which challenges conventional medical paradigms and advocates for patient empowerment. When not producing and directing documentary projects or spearheading initiatives at MS Hope, Mathew enjoys running, reading, music, communing with nature, and spending quality time with his two incredible children. His story of resilience continues to inspire and provide hope to many in their pursuit of optimal health.

Diagnosis Story

It was a day like any other in 1995, marked by the invigorating rush of mountain biking and the joyful simplicity of kicking a ball in my parents' basement. But within moments, everything changed. Suddenly, I couldn't feel the ball the way I normally could.

An unexpected numbness combined with hypersensitivity began to creep up my left side. Initially, I perceived it as an odd sensation, but then the feeling intensified and quickly spread upwards, engulfing my entire left side up to my chest in less than 20 minutes. Before long, my legs began to spasm when I sat.

Assuming I had pinched a nerve during vigorous mountain biking, I initially brushed off the symptoms and waited for them to pass. But when the symptoms persisted for more than a week, my parents and I decided to seek medical attention. After multiple trips to the doctor and an MRI, the verdict finally came from a neurologist, who identified a number of lesions on my brain and spine. The diagnosis was swift and shocking: multiple sclerosis.

I was a 19-year-old athlete at the peak of my physical abilities, with dreams of carving out a career in filmmaking. I envisioned a life of endless possibilities, a life that included a family, full-bodied experiences, and the joy of capturing meaningful stories through my camera lens. But the diagnosis brought my dreams into a harsh confrontation with a new reality.

My understanding of MS was limited, framed by the narratives of comedian Richard Pryor and actress Annette Funicello. Their struggles with the disease painted a future that seemed to hold more despair than hope. My parents and I grappled with the sudden shift in our reality, oscillating between shock and fear. It was hard to believe that this disease had silently infiltrated our lives, threatening to steal my dreams, my mobility, and my freedom.

The diagnosis cast a shadow of uncertainty over my life. The neurologist's words echoed in my mind, "Don't tie concrete blocks to your feet and jump off a bridge just yet." His attempt at injecting a note of grim humor into the situation did little to alleviate my dread. He painted a picture of unpredictability, where the disease could remain a bearable nuisance or transform into a debilitating monster.

As an active 19-year-old, I loved the freedom of movement and using my body. My life was deeply entwined with physical activities: mountain biking, basketball, and filmmaking. The thought of my body betraying me, confining me to a wheelchair, was unthinkable. The prospect of losing my mobility felt akin to losing who I was. I had so many dreams and those dreams included movement and agility.

In those early days, I made a pact with myself. It was a pact born out of fear, despair, and the foolishness of youth. If MS ever reduced me to a life I could not bear, I resolved, that I would end my own life before the disease could rob me of my dignity. A somber choice, yes, but it was a defense mechanism that gave me an odd sense of control over the unpredictable disease. It was my naive way of regaining agency over my own fate: if my life with MS turned out bearable, I'd have a wonderful life, and if it became unbearable, I'd end it on my own terms.

Looking back, I see the flaws in that perspective, but I was just a teenager trying to take control of a life that felt uncontrollable. For me, the MS diagnosis set me apart from my peers, causing an initial sense of alienation. It was hard to reconcile the reality of a chronic illness with the seemingly carefree lives of my friends. The diagnosis forced me to confront the fragility of health and life at an age when most of my contemporaries were exploring their newfound independence and planning their futures.

Fortunately, despite the initial sense of alienation, I found myself surrounded by supportive friends. They became a source of strength and understanding. With their encouragement, I was quickly able to rejoin the crowd and embrace life's joys once again. My friends didn't just provide companionship; they helped me maintain a sense of normalcy, reminding me that while MS was a part of my life, it didn't define my entire existence. It almost never came up in conversation and that is what I preferred. Their support played an integral part in helping me navigate the challenges of living with MS, allowing me to enjoy my youth and live my life to the fullest.

Initially, my diagnosis seemed like a curse, an unwanted interruption in the story of my life. Little did I know that this "curse" would eventually reshape my life in ways I could never imagine. Today, I regard my MS not as a curse, but as a gift, a catalyst for personal growth, and a driving force behind my advocacy work. But that revelation was still years away.

Deciding to Take Care of Myself

Reeling from the shock of the diagnosis, my family and I found ourselves adrift in a sea of uncertainty. We were an ordinary family thrust into what felt like extraordinary circumstances, but we were fortunate. My mother, Joan Embry, was an experienced nurse, and my father, Dr. Ashton Embry, was a research geologist. Their backgrounds in healthcare and research gave us a unique advantage. They knew the grim potential of MS all too well, and their fear became a driving force, propelling them into action.

On the car ride home after the diagnosis, my mother instinctually declared, "This has to have something to do with diet." It was a simple statement, but it was fortuitous.

As soon as the shock of the diagnosis had died down, my father dove headfirst into the medical literature, consuming every piece of information he could find on MS. As he sifted through countless studies and hypotheses, a few serendipitous events spurred us further along our path.

One such event was receiving a book from a teacher from my former high school who was living with MS. The book detailed Dr. Roy Swank's work on how dietary factors, especially consumption of saturated fat, are key contributors to MS. The teacher had adopted Dr. Swank's nutritional recommendations and they were of great benefit for her. As my father's research deepened, he began to see similar patterns. The connections were impossible to ignore.

During this time, pharmaceutical options were limited and largely experimental. Instead of relying solely on these uncertain solutions, my father's research led him to conclude that nutritional changes, high-dose vitamin D, and regular exercise could potentially be key strategies in managing the disease.

From these insights, he formulated the Best Bet Diet: a dietary regimen free from dairy, gluten, and legumes, with low levels of saturated fat and sodium, and generous helpings of vegetables. In many ways, it was very similar to the Paleo diet, which would later gain popularity, and it aligns with what we know today as an anti-inflammatory diet.

The discovery and creation of the Best Bet Diet marked a turning point for our family. We were no longer passive observers in the face of MS; we had armed ourselves with knowledge and were ready to fight back. It felt like we had regained some control in a situation that had initially seemed utterly overwhelming.

My teenage culinary repertoire was dominated by Pizza Pops, chips, cheese, pretzels, Pepsi, and chocolate milk—a dietary lineup that stood in stark contrast to the health-centric principles of the Best Bet Diet. My parents insisted that the entire family adopt this new diet, so our family kitchen transformed into a culinary lab where we experimented with new recipes and cooking techniques that aligned with our new lifestyle. While I admit that a few recipes didn't turn out as expected, I discovered that simplicity in preparation led to better results.

The Tools I Use to Thrive

Personally, I found the transition relatively easy and was excited about adopting a healthier lifestyle. The scientific foundation of the diet instilled confidence in me. I believed firmly that if I adhered to this diet and regular exercise regime, I could hold the reins of my MS. In addition to dietary changes, I also incorporated acupuncture into my regimen, which I felt provided substantial benefits.

I was prescribed a course of steroids immediately after my initial MS attack and this helped alleviate the leg spasms. However, I also experienced adverse side effects from the medication like depression and fatigue. Following that experience, I chose not to use any MS drugs. Instead, I relied on the prescription of diet, exercise, high-dose vitamin D, and the encouragement from stories of people worldwide who had successfully managed their MS symptoms through dietary modifications. Within four to five months of starting the diet and acupuncture, my MS symptoms had completely disappeared.

Our refrigerator door became a billboard for hope, adorned with a printout of Dr. Roy Swank's research as a constant reminder of the crucial role diet played in managing MS. However, this diet-centric approach was met with skepticism and dismissal from the medical community. I recall a follow-up appointment at the MS clinic a few months after I had started the diet. The neurologist was running late, and he casually suggested we have a donut and coffee while waiting. My father and I shared a moment of disbelief; a donut was a confluence of everything the Best Bet Diet advised against—gluten, dairy, high sugar, and fat.

The appointment was a turning point. My father's attempts to discuss the potential of diet in controlling MS were met with disinterest. The neurologist was keen on prescribing pharmaceuticals or having me take part in experimental drug trials, not discussing nutrition. I realized then that my journey to wellness wouldn't be guided by conventional medical practitioners.

Since that day, I have never revisited the MS clinic nor consulted a neurologist for my MS. I chose a different path, one that involved listening to my body, trusting in scientifically backed nutritional strategies, and having faith in my resilience. This road was less travelled and fraught with skepticism. But it was a path that felt instinctively right to me, and it was a path that gave me back control over my life.

I also made the decision to undergo a procedure to address Chronic Cerebrospinal Venous Insufficiency (CCSVI), which is a blood flow issue commonly associated with MS. This treatment is difficult to access due to the controversial nature of its application in MS patients but given the growing body of research suggesting a high association between MS and CCSVI, it felt like a crucial step. Ongoing research gives hope that a deeper understanding of CCSVI could pave the way for innovative treatments for people with MS.

Sharing the Message

Regaining my health and witnessing the effectiveness of the Best Bet Diet instilled in my parents a desire to share their findings with others who were wrestling with MS. My father submitted his Best Bet Diet to the MS Society of Canada, hoping they could distribute this potentially life-altering information to their members. His proposal was met not with interest, however, but apathy. The disinterest from a group dedicated to assisting MS patients was shocking, but we soon realized that the MS Society, neurologists, and the pharmaceutical industry were intricately intertwined.

My parents were faced with a dilemma: they possessed information that could potentially help countless families like ours, yet established channels were closed to them. Undeterred by these roadblocks, my parents took the initiative to start their own charity called Direct-MS in 1996. Direct-MS aimed to share the research my father had gathered about the role of diet and vitamin D in managing MS and to fund research on nutrition and MS.

This initiative was undertaken in the early days of the internet, yet my parents quickly adapted to the digital world. Before the MS Society of Canada even had a website, Direct-MS was online, sharing information with people worldwide. They also took their mission offline, giving talks locally and distributing materials about the Best Bet Diet at health food stores. Through these efforts, they impacted lives both locally and internationally.

Direct-MS began receiving many letters and emails from individuals who had experienced significant health improvements by following the Best Bet Diet. Their efforts to share the diet had borne fruit, improving lives across the globe.

In 2014, I joined my parents' mission to disseminate their valuable insights further. Being a documentary filmmaker, I knew the power of a well-told story. I created the website www.mshope.com to share information about MS in a user-friendly, accessible way, and in multiple languages. The website reached many thousands of people worldwide, with countless messages flooding in, more than I could ever keep up with.

Wanting to amplify our message even further, I started filming a documentary called *Living Proof*. This project was an opportunity to capture our family's journey and inspire hope in others facing similar challenges. *Living Proof* premiered at the Toronto International Film Festival in 2017 and is now globally distributed on Amazon Prime in multiple languages.

Living Proof: Impact and Advocacy

For me, *Living Proof* was more than just a film; it was a powerful tool to share our message of resilience, exploration, and hope. The response from the MS community and the wider audience was overwhelming. The documentary resonated with people across the globe, many of whom had been searching for alternative ways to manage their MS symptoms. It brought our family's story to an international audience, shining a light on the potential role of diet in managing MS. Additionally, I had the privilege of sharing in the film the inspiring stories of individuals who had achieved remarkable healing and recovery.

The film propelled me into a role I hadn't initially sought but quickly embraced: that of an advocate for people with MS. As *Living Proof* gained traction, it opened platforms for me to engage with audiences on a broader scale all over the world. I was able to share not only my personal journey but also share the scientific information that had formed our approach to managing MS.

Being an advocate means that I can offer a different perspective to those diagnosed with MS. The conventional prognosis often paints a bleak picture, one filled with disability and despair. However, my experience has shown me that alternative routes exist, and they can lead to health and empowerment. It was a message I felt compelled to share, providing a counternarrative to the often-doom-laden prognosis of MS.

Mindset Work

Today, I view my MS not as a debilitating disease but as an integral part of my journey. It has shaped me, driven me, and inspired me to help others facing similar challenges. Despite its difficulties, I wouldn't change my journey with MS. It has taught me resilience, opened my eyes to the power of advocating for oneself, and showed me that hope is a key ingredient in the face of adversity.

As I reflect on my journey with MS, I can say with confidence that I'm living an incredible life. I have a fulfilling career as a filmmaker and engage in marathons and trail races. I am blessed with two wonderful teenagers, supported by my loving wife Eun Jung Lee, and completely free of MS symptoms. I wholeheartedly attribute my well-being to the Best Bet Diet, daily exercise, high-dose vitamin D, mindfulness practices, and the positive, inspiring people in my life.

However, the true significance of my story is not in the telling but in its potential to benefit you. It's my hope that by sharing my experience, you can gain insight, feel inspired, and perhaps consider new possibilities for managing your health, especially if you're dealing with MS.

It's essential to note that my approach isn't a quick fix or an easy route. There are no cheat days. If you want to see results, commitment is crucial. Half measures yield half the benefits. Maintaining the Best Bet Diet and lifestyle regimen requires discipline, but from my perspective, the rewards are unparalleled.

At the end of the day, we're all allotted a limited amount of time on this planet. My family's mission and mine is to make the absolute best of that time, and we want to help others do the same. We aim to provide information that can help optimize your health and enhance your experience as a human, whether or not you have MS.

Remember, the choice is entirely yours. Your journey is unique, and only you can decide the path that feels right. Whatever your decision, know that there are options, there is hope, and there is the potential for an abundant, healthy life.

4

Multiple Sclerosis Is My Sidekick

Robyn Pineault

Persistence and resilience only come from having been given the chance to work through difficult problems.

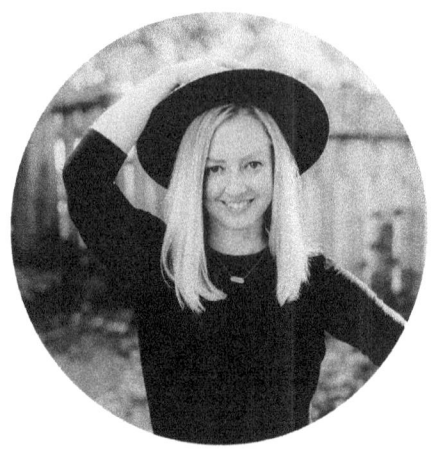

ROBYN PINEAULT

Robyn Pineault is an MS Thriver. Her mission in life is to empower those living with an autoimmune disease to thrive and not just survive. Robyn lives in Ottawa with her husband, twin toddlers and 2 fur babies. She is a Marketing Director, a health & lifestyle blogger at RobynPineault.com, the author of Love Lost, Life Found, the former podcast host of The Alpha Female Podcast and a passionate Essential Oil Educator. She loves weightlifting, yoga, outdoor adventures (from hiking to canoe trips) and making seasonal bucket lists. You can follow her on Instagram at @robynpineault for more tips on thriving with an autoimmune disease.

Diagnosis Story

The moment the doctor said, "There is an abnormality on the MRI," my world stopped for a split second. The next words out of his mouth were, "There is demyelination on the C spine, which is indicative of MS but not conclusive."

It's indicative but not conclusive?! I thought. *Do you think you could figure things out and give me a more definite answer before you change my entire world!!?!!*

Let me back up for a second. I woke up Tuesday, November 25, 2014, with numb, tingling fingers in my right hand. I thought I had slept funny on my arm and my fingers were simply asleep. I was a gym rat back then, so I packed my gym and food bag and headed off to the gym before work. I went through a back workout, stretched, foam rolled, and lay on a ball under my scapula & traps thinking I had a pinched nerve somewhere in my neck. Throughout the day my upper torso (major pec/boob) went numb and then my abs and back down my right side. Finally, when the numbness and tingling had reached all the way down my right leg within a week, I drove myself to the hospital, where I received a CAT scan and two

MRIs before a definitive diagnosis—clinically isolated multiple sclerosis—was proclaimed by a neurologist.

Over the course of my time in the hospital and the days after diagnosis, I went into action mode. I posted about my diagnosis. I asked for help and resources and boy, did I get them. And I'm thankful that I did. Over the next few months, I started sorting through all the recommendations so I could do my own research.

Deciding to Take Care of Myself

From the time I announced my diagnosis, I began to witness different reactions. There were the opinion / advice givers. It can be overwhelming, but if you sort through the gamut of resources offered you might just find something that works for you. There were the practical help offers. These were invaluable, like people offering to help me with grocery shopping, etc. These are true friends that go above and beyond the "let me know how I can help" offers. There were the people who echoed back exactly what I needed to hear and became my cheerleaders, and then there were the "woe is me" reactions.

These were the ones where I saw pity in their eyes or in their words on social media. As they told me "I'm so sorry," I came to learn that most people say that to follow societal niceties. And when I thought about it a little more, I realized that most people put themselves in your shoes and can't imagine what it would be like to live with a health diagnosis such as MS, so they simply say, "I'm so sorry." Because, in reality, they would be feeling sorry if it had happened to them.

I never wanted to experience pity again, so I knew I had to figure out how to take care of myself so this disease would never decrease the quality of my life. I'm determined to not let this disease shorten my life span, and I want a thriving health span so that I can enjoy all the moments of my life. Even up until my last days.

Living with an autoimmune disease can be challenging and unpredictable. Managing symptoms, ensuring symptoms never pop up, navigating medical appointments, and more requires resilience, patience, grace, and the ability to constantly adapt.

I decided to overhaul my life, from nutrition to supplementation to sleep to stress management to reducing my toxic load (more about that later). And it was working. I even boldly wrote a blog post three years after my diagnosis proclaiming my MS to be in remission. I was confident with how I took care of myself and that this "health sidekick," as I called it, was never going to get the better of me.

Fast forward to 2023, and after years of being flare free, I woke up on February 14th to my first MS attack in nine years. But this time, there was no doctor to misuse words and confuse me. I went to see my family doctor and requested to be seen again by the Ottawa MS Clinic. In 2016, I had actually stopped going to see my neurologist at the MS Clinic because I refused to go on disease-modifying drugs so they said there was nothing they could do for me. So back to this year... I had two new MRI scans done. When I got access to my new MRI results and could clearly read that I had one lesion on my spine (the original culprit), I knew this was the cause of the current numbness and tingling on my right side. The year after my diagnosis, that lesion appeared smaller, which I attribute to all the things I did to reduce inflammation in my body.

To be completely honest, I spent the next few months beating myself up. *I thought you had this figured out. What did you do or not do to develop a flare?* and more self-talk that was less than supportive. But I came to realize I was simply coasting along. I wasn't diving into new research to see what else my health sidekick might have to teach me. So, I started digging around again, just like I did when I was first diagnosed. One of the articles that caught my attention was published in January 2022 in Science magazine[3].

I learned that as early as 2011, studies have found evidence suggesting that those with MS are more likely to have been exposed to the Epstein-Barr virus (EBV) in their lifetime and that the virus may trigger the autoimmune response that leads to the development of MS[4]. One study

---

[3] Bjornevik, K., et al. (2022). Longitudinal analysis reveals high prevalence of Epstein-Barr virus associated with multiple sclerosis. *Science* 375(6578): 296–301.
https://www.science.org/doi/10.1126/science.abj8222

[4] Pender, M. P. (2011). The essential role of Epstein-Barr virus in the pathogenesis of multiple sclerosis. Neuroscientist 17(4): 351–67.
https://doi.org/10.1177/1073858410381531
Sundqvist, E., et al. (2012). Epstein-Barr virus and multiple sclerosis: interaction with HLA. Genes and Immunity 13(1): 14–20. https://doi.org/10.1038/gene.2011.42
Lunemann, J. D., et al. (2018). Epstein-Barr virus as a trigger of autoimmune diseases. Best Practice & Research Clinical Rheumatology 32(2): 185–96.
https://doi.org/10.1016/j.berh.2018.10.006
Serafini, B., et al. (2019). Epstein-Barr virus latent membrane protein 1 triggers a pro-inflammatory cytokine cascade in multiple sclerosis brain. Journal of Neuroinflammation 16(1): 14.
https://doi.org/10.1186/s12974-019-1394-4
Marrodán, M., et al. (2021). Early Epstein-Barr virus infection and multiple sclerosis: a systematic review and meta-analysis. Multiple

found that individuals who were infected with EBV at a young age had a higher risk of developing MS later in life, while another study found that levels of certain antibodies produced in response to EBV were higher in people with MS than in those without the disease. Another study found that a specific protein produced by EBV can activate immune cells that attack the myelin sheath that surrounds nerve cells, leading to the symptoms of MS. That Science article included information about new treatments that deplete the body of B cells containing the EBV virus.

This MS flare is teaching me that I do still have more to learn about this health sidekick and that there are things I can do to thrive again.

The Tools I Use to Thrive

Here are all the things that I learned and did to keep me symptom-free for nine years—and that I'm continuing to do as I navigate my first flare.

Sclerosis and Related Disorders 51: 102875. https://doi.org/10.1016/j.msard.2021.102875

The Six Pillars of Health

I believe that we can optimize our life so that our body's cells don't get confused and attack us. This is possible by focusing on what I call the six pillars of health.

The Six Pillars of Health:
- Nutrition
- Supplements
- Movement/exercise
- Sleep
- Stress management
- Reduce toxic load

After getting several requests from friends to chat with someone they know who is newly diagnosed with MS, I created an Autoimmune Healing Guide that I give away for free on my website.

In the guide, I ask those who download it to write down the six pillars and rank them from 1 to 5, with 1 being you don't know a lot about optimizing this area of your life and 5 being you've got this area of your life under control. From there I share book and podcast recommendations that have served me well, and then I ask lots of questions to get you to think about where to focus your attention, research, and resources.

My top three books that I read when I was diagnosed were The Autoimmune Solution by Amy Myers, M.D., The Autoimmune Wellness Handbook by Mickey Trescott and Angie Alt, and Your Longevity Blueprint by Dr. Stephanie Gray.

The top three podcasts that I enjoyed listening to were The Autoimmune Wellness Podcast and The Ultimate Health Podcast.

Here are several things related to each pillar that I did/do to thrive.

Nutrition

The diet that works best may be different for everyone. I researched the Wahls Protocol, the AIP Protocol, the Swank Diet, and the Best Bet Diet and found that for me, the AIP Protocol and elimination diet was most successful at healing my leaky gut at the time of my diagnosis. Things that I'm looking into now around nutrition involve looking at my bloodwork regularly to see what vitamins and minerals I may be deficient in. I always want to optimize my nutrition before I supplement to solve deficiencies. In addition, I'm looking at what root cause could be causing a deficiency. With nutrition and supplementation changes, I consider these to be short-term band-aid solutions and until you figure out the root cause making these changes long-term isn't always sustainable. Once you've discovered and addressed the root cause of many digestive issues like parasites, mold exposure, candida or SIBO (as examples), long-term elimination diets might no longer be needed.

Supplements

I have always worked with a naturopath to optimize my supplementation protocol based on bloodwork results. A supplementation protocol will look different for everyone. When I'm building a healthcare team, I always try to bring them one or two objectives that I'd like to work on solving. This will help focus them on their supplement recommendations. Example: 1. Reduce inflammation; 2. Increase energy.

I also work with practitioners who will make nutrition recommendations before prescribing supplements. However, with the quality of food and nutrients in the earth severely lacking these days, supplementation is of course necessary.

In addition, once supplements have been recommended, I then begin researching the companies that are being recommended. Unfortunately, the supplement industry is not regulated, and we do need to be careful that the supplements we are taking actually contain the necessary therapeutic dosages that will support our bodies. When working with a healthcare team, always discuss the appropriate times to recheck blood work after being put on a protocol.

Movement/Exercise

While my first year after diagnosis was spent proving that I was stronger than MS by running over 20 obstacle course races, I put myself into adrenal fatigue and have learned that less is more when it comes to MS. While staying consistently active is important, I'm no longer pushing myself to extremes. My body thrives with 20-to-30-minute bodyweight or light resistance workouts three to four times a week and yoga once a week. I also take a walk every morning with my husband and our two dogs.

Sleep

I focused/focus (it's an ongoing process) on getting a quality eight hours of sleep a night. This includes a relaxing evening routine.

I have found that I need to be truly religious with my evening routine to get a great night's sleep. That includes spending time winding down after we put our twins to bed at 7:30 pm. Usually 2–3 times a week I take an Epsom salt bath with Borax powder (I have a boron deficiency). On the other nights, I am running a detox program in our infrared sauna where I'll spend at least 30 to 45 minutes. On the one night when I'm heading off to a hot yoga class, I'll take a cold shower afterwards before crawling into bed.

In addition to baths, saunas and showers, I have set up a plug timer to turn off our Wi-Fi at 10 pm and then turn it back on at 5 am. I'm trying to be strict and not allow myself any screen time for at least an hour before bed, so I'll plug in my phone in our bathroom and then I'll crawl into bed with a book. I use a Hatch alarm clock with a light and have programmed it with a wind-down routine; when I crawl into bed I'll hit the top and it'll start Stage 1, which is 30 minutes of bright light so I can read, and then it'll switch to Stage 2, where the light gets dimmer and signals for me to put my book away and get ready for sleep. It'll go for 10 minutes before switching off completely.

Stress Management

I focus on proactive and reactive stress management. While my evening routine helps set me up for sleep, it also helps me wind down from the stress of the day. In regard to proactive stress management, I know that when I stick to a great morning routine I'm much more likely to be able to face daily stress in a much better way.

When I open my eyes, I pop into the bathroom to empty my bladder, then I'll tongue scrape and oil pull. From there I'll head to the kitchen to make warm lemon water with Redmond salt and a small spoonful of honey. Then I move to my home office for meditation, red light therapy, journaling, and/or prayer.

I've been experimenting with cold plunges and have been trying to get at least three mins 2–3 times a week. I usually do these in the mornings on the days I'm having a shower so I'll cold plunge (by filling up my bathtub with cold water and adding ice), shower, and then get ready for my workday.

Finally, I'm a huge fan of doing talk therapy, ensuring I have at least one monthly date with a friend, planning weekly date nights with my husband, and attempting to read some fiction since I'm usually nose deep in nonfiction.

Reduce Toxic Load

Earlier in the chapter I talked about creating an environment where my body couldn't get confused. To accomplish this, it's imperative to reduce the toxic load in my body. Unfortunately, toxins are everywhere, and we won't be able to avoid them completely unless we decide to live in a bubble, but there are so many things we can proactively do to reduce the toxic load on our bodies.

For example, I've switched out all my cleaning and beauty products for ones that have a more natural ingredient list, or I make my own with essential oils. I removed anything from my home that has known endocrine disruptors, including beauty products and makeup. I avoid touching receipts and drinking my decaf coffee from to-go containers. My whole family and I do a hard-metal detox several times a year. We buy organic produce as much as possible and I support local regenerative farmers by purchasing pasture-raised, grass-fed, and grass-finished meat. I've even learned how to hunt so I can "hopefully" fill the freezer with game meat in the future.

Finally, I'm taking time to truly research the impact that parasites might have on my health. I'm looking into working with knowledgeable practitioners, testing and then learning how to treat them appropriately to support my overall health.

Mindset Work

While optimizing and/or overhauling the six pillars of health there is one more thing to focus on in parallel. This is where mindset work comes into play.

When facing a major health diagnosis, most of us will go through grief, and supporting ourselves through that grief will be individualized. When I was diagnosed, I was aware of the five stages of grief, but I wanted to jump straight to acceptance. But I've since learned that processing grief is not linear. You don't always move directly from one stage to the next. I like to describe processing grief as a game of Whac-A-Mole. One day you might deal with anger, and then another day you'll deal with sadness, and then acceptance, and then back to denial or anger. Once you recognize what stage you're in at any given time, you can reach for the tools to support yourself.

Because I went straight to acceptance and learning to live with MS, I ignored the fact that I needed to grieve my former self. I experienced an identity death and rebirth, and I hadn't properly felt all my feelings around that. It wasn't until the MS flare occurred in 2023 that I truly dealt with sadness, wrestled with a lot of feelings, and asked myself a lot of questions. For example:

What if my life doesn't return to normal?
What if my life expectancy is shortened?
What if I die young?
What if I must use a wheelchair?
What if I can't pick up my twins?

And while I needed to go to the depths of darkness, I also needed to give myself a hand and pull myself out of the hole that I was crawling into. I needed to accept what currently is but also acknowledge that I'm not in darkness. I am not physically disabled. I have figured this out before, and I can figure it out again. And if I can't, I have an immense support system around me that will support me regardless of my physical capabilities.

My Health Sidekick

Robin to Batman.
Tonto to the Lone Ranger.
Mini-Me to Dr. Evil.
Chewbacca to Han Solo.

It seems like every hero has a sidekick. But how do sidekicks relate to living with MS?

When diagnosed with a disease, instead of thinking of ourselves as "living with MS" we might take on an identity associated with the disease such as "MS Warrior," "MSer," "MS Advocate," "MS Fighter," or "MS Survivor." Hell, I've used them myself. I even use "MS Thriver" or "Autoimmune Thriver" to ensure I'm having a positive identity birth after the diagnosis. But because my life seemed consumed with living with MS when I was first diagnosed, I really didn't want to lose myself in the disease.

So, I decided to perceive MS not as something to fight against, or a persona to take on, but rather as an unconventional type of sidekick. In many cases, a sidekick is there to support the hero, watch their back, keep them honest, and so on. I see my "health sidekick" as an unexpected hitchhiker that you pick up for a long road trip across the country. That sidekick might not always be supportive; they might require you to adapt and grow. They might teach you patience. They might remind you that you haven't been on top of your self-care as well as you could be.

Becoming highly attuned to my body through self-awareness and self-compassion is what my health sidekick has taught me. Calling it a sidekick was imperative for me to stop viewing myself as someone with a disease and rather as someone who simply lives well because her sidekick reminds her to take care of herself.

It's Not a Death Sentence

The final mindset shift that was important for me to work on was not viewing the diagnosis as a death sentence. I had to learn to ignore people like the neurologist who mentioned that my lifespan might be shorter than before and my boyfriend at the time of my diagnosis who broke up with me because he feared me having to use a wheelchair in the future. I made the decision early on that I was going to live a great life with MS as my sidekick and that I did not have to fear death. And having a supportive husband who tells you he'll support you no matter what lies ahead in our road. So when my life does end, I will have chosen to nurture the quality of my life to the best of my ability all along the way.

5

Strength In Faith

Sara Stewart

Resilience is weathering the storm of life and coming out the other side stronger.

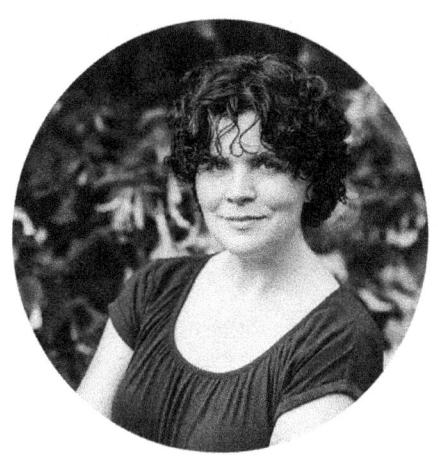

SARA STEWART

Sara Stewart is a mother of three, wife of almost 20 years, sister and friend. She lives in a small town in southern Manitoba where she and her family have resided for almost 15 years. Before her diagnosis, she was a realtor and now works for Canada Post. In her spare time, she enjoys gardening, spending time with family at their cottage, walking her two adorable Bernedoodles and running her kids to all their hockey, lacrosse and gymnastic practices. Sara has a strong Christian faith and attends Be The Church Fellowship in Winnipeg, MB. She is open to sharing about her struggles with MS and how she was able to overcome the hardships of her diagnosis and disease. She has found success in holistic practices that have given her a new passion for health and wellness.

Diagnosis Story

What was supposed to be a normal Saturday morning getting our two young boys ready for a hockey tournament turned out to change me and my family's lives forever.

The alarm clock woke me up at 5:30 am and I went down to the basement where we had a makeshift kitchen since we were undergoing a total kitchen renovation. I quickly made something for the boys to eat in the car for breakfast since we were already running behind schedule. I was standing on the cement floor and noticed I could feel the cold on one foot and nothing on the other one. I thought it was weird, but I didn't have time to give it much thought. I finished breakfast, packed up the boys, and we took off for the hockey tournament.

During the first game, I noticed that the leg of the foot that couldn't feel the cold was now feeling hot from my knee down. My mind went right to the thought of it being a blood clot, even though I knew that wasn't it. I asked some of the moms if I should be worried and they told me to just watch it. After the game, I went to the bathroom. My hand touched my skin under my shirt and instantly I was in tears. It felt like I had just electrocuted myself.

What's going on? This isn't normal. I walked out and my friend asked me what happened. I told her I needed to go to the ER right away. My husband stayed with the boys and my friend took me to the hospital, where I told her I would be fine, and she should head back to the hockey rink. I would call my husband, Brian, with updates. I was brought back into the examining room where the doctor asked lots of questions, poked me with many different things to see what would give me the electric shock feeling, and stood around very puzzled. After being there for the whole day and into the evening I asked one of the nurses, "If I am not dying can I please go to the evening hockey game?" As much as I had loved spending the day with them, I wanted to see my son's evening game. They told me they had to run one more test and if it came back normal, I could go. So, I waited and waited, then was told that everything came back normal, and they had no clue why I was getting these feelings when objects would come into contact with my skin. They advised me to make an appointment with my family doctor on Monday and sent me on my way.

First thing Monday morning, I said goodbye to the kids, kissed my husband, and headed off to another ER in Winnipeg as advised by my sister who is an ICU nurse. I got there, checked in, and the wait began. I waited and waited and waited. After 12 hours of waiting, I was finally brought back to the examining area where of course I waited some more. Finally, a doctor came in and I told her everything that had happened. She started to examine me but by this time my body was so used to having things being put onto it that hurt, I would start to flinch without even noticing. She told me she was just going to try some ice and see how it felt. I don't remember ever having pain like that. Tears just ran down my face. All I could do was ask her to please stop. She informed me she was going to talk to the neurologist and find out if he wanted to see me.

After a little break from the doctor and supper from my sister, the neurologist asked me questions. At one point he asked me if anyone in my family had multiple sclerosis and I said no one did, but in my mind, I was like, *that was a weird question*. You can't just wake up one day after being totally fine and then have MS. The truth was I didn't know much about MS, but in due time that would change.

Once all the questions were asked, he told me I needed an MRI and that someone would come grab me once they were ready. My sister said her goodbyes and told me my dad was on the way to be with me for the MRI and whatever was to come after that. In no time I was wheeled to the MRI area. At this time, I was a little unsure about what was going to happen; I didn't know what an MRI machine looked like or really what it did. They asked me if I was claustrophobic and I said, "I don't think so," but boy was I wrong. I was transferred to the bed and given earplugs, headphones, and a little ball to squeeze if I wasn't okay. I started to be moved into the machine and as I went farther and farther into it, I thought to myself, Will this ever end? I know it's not that long and that there is an opening on the other side, but when you are in there it feels so long and that is when I figured out, I was claustrophobic. My mind was everywhere and nowhere at the same time. I had no clue what was going on. I cried the whole time. All I knew was it wasn't good if they were doing all these tests so quickly.

Once the MRI was done, they wheeled me back into the ER triage area where my dad was waiting. We sat there listening to the hockey game on the radio and waited to find out what was next. The neurologist came to see us and told us that there was no active lesion on my spine. There was an old mark, but he didn't feel like it was important, maybe an old injury had caused that mark, he told me. The game plan from here was to come back and do a brain MRI because they had only done the spine. I was told his office would be in touch and I could go home. Over 12 hours of sitting and waiting just to leave with more questions than answers. *Why had they asked about MS, what was MS, and how could I just wake up one morning and have it?*

The next couple of days things did not get better. Sitting on the toilet was getting more and more painful, having showers was a no-go, and I was still not sure why my body felt this way. At this point, I was not scared or even worried, but more annoyed. On Wednesday, I was taking my youngest son to the city for his hockey skate and was not able to tie his skates. My hands just could not grab the lace and tie it up. At this point, I was so scared. My husband worked away from home; if I could not use my hands, how could I take care of my boys and myself?

On the way home, I received a call from an MRI technician who asked me if I could come in that evening because they had just had a cancellation. I said yes immediately, and she asked me if my symptoms were getting worse. I told her what had happened at hockey, and she said she was happy that I was able to make the appointment. So that evening I went back into the MRI machine but this time with a cage over my head, the same loud noise, tears running down my face, and me just singing "Jesus Loves Me" over and over again. How could life have changed so fast in such a short time?

It was not long before reality came smacking me in the face. That Friday, I was called to head to the hospital where my uncle was dying from pancreatic cancer, and they thought he was not going to last much longer. It was a hard day, not sure what was happening and seeing my uncle. He asked me how I was doing and told me he wished that I was not suffering so much. I told him that I would stay strong just like he had done through these past months. My phone rang and I told him I would be right back. The call was from the neurologist. He apologized for calling so late on Friday and asked if things were getting better. I told him they were the same and he said he was not surprised since the MRI results showed that my brain was a mess. *What did that mean, why was it a mess?* He told me that I needed to start taking steroids right away and to see him in his office in two and a half weeks. I asked what was causing the issues with my brain and all of the symptoms and that was the first time he said they were considering MS. I thanked him and my only thoughts were, *at least I am not dying and can see my kids grow up.* Life will be hard, but I can still be here for them.

Deciding to Take Care of Myself

Over the next two and a half weeks I did a deep dive on the internet, trying to figure out what I had, whether it was really MS, and if so, how I could make it better. Did I have options or was this a slow death sentence? Right then, I decided that if I had it and there was something I could do to feel better, I would do it. While searching online I came across two websites that gave me so much hope. One was from a lady in the United Kingdom, and another was from a gentleman here in Canada. Both had been living with MS for a long time and both were doing very well managing their disease. I had to know what they had done, and I was determined to follow their lifestyles so I could have the best life possible even though I now had this incurable disease.

Two and a half weeks later, I was back in the doctor's office to hear what they had to say. They had me fill out so much paperwork and do a bunch of tests, like making me walk as fast as I could and timing me, and a peg test (you had to use one hand to take a peg out of a bowl and put it into a hole, then do it with the other hand). My husband had found this all so weird and asked the doctor right when he came in why I had to do all these tests and he said, "Well, she has MS, relapsing and remitting, and this is how we track how her body is changing." Right then and there: "She has MS." To the doctor, it seemed like no big deal, but to me, my life would never be the same. The rest of the appointment was a blur. I never cried, I was not mad, there were just a lot of unknowns. They told me they would see me in six weeks to talk about drug options. I already knew that was not the way I wanted to go. All the reading I'd done had shown me that the drugs did not stop the MS; at best they stopped the attacks by 30%. Yes, only 30%. I had made the decision that if the drugs could not stop the progression of the MS, I was not going to take them. This led to many doctor appointments, and I fought to stand my ground on this. This was my life, not theirs, and I wanted the best chance to have a normal life. Over time I told my doctor that we would agree to disagree on this matter.

I was learning that diet and exercise could help more than drugs. But it was going to be hard. With two young boys, how was I going to do this? The first step that I took was to book an appointment with a naturopathic doctor who would support my journey of avoiding drugs and pursuing more natural treatment options. We started off by doing an E95 Common Food Panel, which tests for sensitivity to foods because managing MS is about managing inflammation. This was the first step to see what foods I reacted to at the blood level. While we waited for that test to come back, I started the Autoimmune Elimination Diet. This was one of the hardest things I have ever tried. I felt like there was not really anything I could eat. Food became something I ate to help heal my body, but I did not enjoy it like I had before. Food had always been about family and celebration and now it was neither of those things. It was work. Once the food panel results came back, I started making other dietary changes (more on that later).

Months passed and I was settling into my new life managing the symptoms that had become my new norm, when things drastically changed again, this time for a new family member: I was pregnant. I was shocked and not sure how I would manage. I was constantly tired and had never felt like that before. I would get up with the boys, get them to school, and come home and sleep all day. I just remember thinking, I cannot live life like this. Is this how it's going to be? I was told that I should be fine and that most women with MS do well with pregnancy. The only risk factor was that for three months after the baby was born, I would be at an 80% increased risk of a relapse. The first three months of pregnancy were tough. Morning sickness was brutal until my naturopath told me about acupuncture. I started right away, and it was a game-changer for me; it's a tool that I still use to this day. Once the third trimester came, I was feeling great. I felt like my old self before I was diagnosed with MS.

Almost a year after I was diagnosed with MS, we welcomed our daughter into the world. And just like the doctors had warned me, around the three-month mark I had a relapse that would last weeks. At this point, I had learned a lot and with the help of my naturopath, we got to the other side of it. Along the way, I was finding new tools that would help when things started to act up and my symptoms worsened. These tools were IV therapy, extra supplementations and stress management practice.

Fast forward 7 years to the summer of 2021, when I was given the COVID-19 vaccine, and it sent my MS into a flare that I could not get under control. I was given steroids to calm things down, but it just made me feel worse. I was trying more natural treatments with some success, but nothing was really giving long-term relief. I dove deeper into the internet and researched what treatments were showing good results on halting MS. I found a procedure called hematopoietic stem cell transplant, or HSCT, that had good results and was available here in Canada. However, I very quickly realized I would not be considered for it because you had to fail on two of the disease-modifying drugs before they would put you on the waitlist. So back I went to the internet, where I found that it was also being done in Mexico at a private state-of-the-art clinic.

I started praying for clear signs that this was what I should do, and I felt like every door that I had to walk through was opening. Throughout this process, I had to trust, and I leaned on my faith to direct me when I was unsure of the next step. The results of HSCT are very good and this clinic had good reviews, so together with my husband and my family we made the decision that I was going to go. This was not an easy decision as it meant I would be away for a month and leaving my kids for that long was going to be so hard. Everyone was going to have to step up to help. My oldest sister, the nurse, took time off from work to be with me the whole time. My parents were on call just in case my husband had to go back to work. My daughter's birthday was planned months in advance so that it would be easy for my husband to handle it while I was away. Everything worked out so smoothly and I was so thankful that I could focus on my treatment and recovery and trust that everything else was taken care of by my family, who had supported me this entire time.

Recovery has been long and frustrating at times, but day by day things do get easier. It's always a journey of two steps forward and one step back, still always moving forward. After the HSCT treatment, I started walking my two dogs to build up my cardio; at first, it was a block at a time, and I have now built up to six miles a day. My strength has improved as well. I can do HIIT classes without my MS starting to act up. This was so great to see because I had not been able to do high-intensity workouts since a few years after being diagnosed. My most recent MRI showed no new lesions and some of my old lesions decreased in size or were not there anymore. This in itself is a success that I do not take for granted and I give thanks to God every day.

The Tools I Use to Thrive

As I move forward and try to do as much as I can to care for myself, naturally I have to look back and see what has worked and not worked for me. Just like MS is different for everyone, everyone's body will respond differently to treatment. I have found that I need to blend a little bit of knowledge and tips from one source and a little bit from another source to find my optimal health. There really isn't any one diet or one set of guidelines that worked for me. Realizing this helped me start discovering the direction I needed to go in. It has not been a straight line; rather, it has been a journey full of curves and ever-changing directions, but I have identified key areas that I will always focus on.

Naturopathic Medicine

Naturopathic medicine has been a central pillar of my treatment journey. The E95 Common Food Panel I mentioned earlier was a very important starting point. It provided an outline of a healthy diet for me and my specific situation and detailed what I needed to remove from my diet to minimize the inflammatory process that was driving my symptoms.

I also learned about taking supplements to supply important nutrients, like vitamin B12 and vitamin D. Maintaining adequate levels of vitamin B12 has always been hard for me, though, so instead of supplementing in pill form I needed to get a shot every two weeks. As for vitamin D, I increase my levels via supplements in different seasons but try as much as I can to be out in the sun without sunscreen for about 15 minutes a day, especially in the summer months. As for other supplements, those change depending on how my body is feeling; this is why working with a naturopathic doctor was so important for managing my disease. A unique treatment we tried with some success when I had minor flares in the past was 10-pass ozone therapy, where your blood is mixed with ozone in a bottle and then put back into your body intravenously.

Gut Health

One of the first things that needs to be prioritized when diagnosed is to work on building a healthy gut. Leaky gut is known to have a role in the development of MS and it's important to heal it and to support it moving forward. To support good digestion and a healthy gut microbiome, I make sure to take a good pre/probiotic, switching them up every so often because different brands have different strains of bacteria in them. I incorporate fermented foods and drinks into my diet, limit sugar intake, and stay away from foods I have a sensitivity to.

Toxin Load

I learned that it is important to lower the toxins you come into contact with, whether in your house or the products you use on your body. I have removed toxic products and incorporated non-toxic organic versions as well as essential oils into my home. I use essential oils in hand soap, cleaning supplies, laundry soap, dryer balls, and in diffusers around my home. I buy products like shampoo and conditioner that contain essential oils and I even make my own face and body lotion. They work great to repel ticks, mosquitoes, or any bug that is a nuisance outdoors.

Healthy Eating

This is an area where I always feel like I could do better. I don't know if I will ever be where I "should" be, but I will keep moving forward. Once I knew the results of the E95 Common Food Panel, my diet started changing. I have stayed away from gluten, dairy, eggs, and legumes and increased my vegetables and proteins. I eat lots of wild meat as well as salmon. Both fish oils and flaxseed oils have become a staple in my diet. Cutting back on sugar has been hard but is needed. Limiting processed food is important, so I now cook at home on a daily basis. I have found websites with recipes for people who have dietary restrictions and I have learned how to substitute ingredients in recipes to fit my diet and improve the nutritional value.

Holistic Nutritionist

From the beginning of my journey with MS, I have discovered what I eat and how I supplement vitamins and minerals to be the most important aspect of treatment I can control. My sister and I have always connected in this way and continue to share ideas and support for each other's health and wellness. Since my diagnosis, my sister has decided to pursue a career in holistic nutrition and wants to help support others with diseases like MS to live their best lives. The hope is that this information will offer prevention and/or treatment to those in our family and community.

Exercise

This has changed over the eight years since my diagnosis, and I expect that it will continue to change as I get older. To me, it is important to at least walk my dogs once a day for both the physical and mental benefits. Weight training is also important for staying healthy, regardless of the fact that I have an autoimmune disease. I have realized that it is important to listen to my body; it will tell me what it can handle and what it does not like. I have found that doing low-impact exercise has better results for my body than high-impact exercise.

Stress Reduction

I have learned over the years that I cannot dwell on things that I cannot change and to not get too upset over things. This hasn't been easy, but once I understood that the stress it causes was hurting me, I made the decision to let things go and move on. Acupuncture has been a good tool for managing my stress when it gets too high due to situations out of my control. I have also focused on meditation and prayer when feeling overwhelmed.

Frequency Therapy

Frequency therapy uses vibrational frequencies to heal the body at the cellular level. This is not a new technique; it has been around since the 1900s, fell out of use in the 1940s, then came back into popularity in the 1980s. I have not been able to see the benefits yet as I have only done it for the past few months, but I am always learning and open to trying new things to better care for my health as I age.

Gardening

This has become such a passion for me. Gardening helps with my stress levels, gets me outside in nature, and provides me with fresh vegetables and herbs. When I can fuel myself with food that does not have pesticides on it and is grown in my backyard, I feel so much better about what I am putting in my body.

Mindset Work

My faith and belief in God is the most important thing in my life and gets me through tough times, but it also makes me so grateful for the life I have been given. I have been blessed with the most amazing family that has been on this journey with me for the last eight years and together we have grown so much that I don't know if I could have made it this far without them. This journey has been both mentally and physically challenging, but I know with them by my side I can face anything. We do not know where this journey will go but I feel like I have some control over the direction by choosing the disciplined, natural way and fighting it head-on. I trust that I was given this diagnosis for a reason and I'm going to try my hardest to support others in similar situations while keeping a positive attitude.

6

Trusting Your Intuition Through Illness

Sarah St. John

Resilience is the ability to adapt, persevere, commit, and even flourish amidst challenges and adversity. Like the flower that grows in the crack of the pavement, it brings hope.

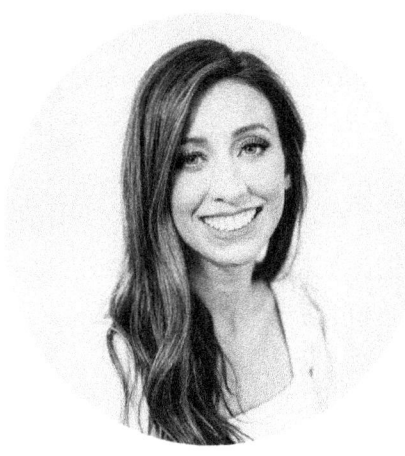

SARAH ST. JOHN

Sarah St. John is a mama of 2, entrepreneur, podcaster, and author. As a 13+ year teacher and mentor, she supports creative & neurodivergent empaths to use their story to breathe life back into people. Through her company, The Uncensored Empath LLC, Sarah has coached thousands of women to get back in their bodies and feel again. She is well-versed in navigating the hardest in-between spaces in life and uses tools such as somatic experiencing, breathwork, yoga, tapping, and nervous system healing to help her clients leave a creative legacy they are proud of. For empath tips & lots of emotion-based storytelling follow Sarah on Instagram at @sarahsaintjohn.

Diagnosis Story

I walked into a hot yoga studio just a few months before I graduated college.

I thought it would be a fun workout with my girlfriends. But instead of just sweating out the four years of beer drinking and late-night partying, I sweat out all my body dissociation. And now it was clear: I was not well.

The clues began in middle school when, shortly after my parents got divorced, I wound up in the hospital with severe abdominal pain and was eventually diagnosed with stomach migraines. These would come and go throughout my youth, but at their worst, they would jolt me out of a deep sleep and the only thing that would bring relief was a hot bath in the middle of the night.

The thing about not learning how to be "in" your body as a child is you don't develop a sense of normal, or even what feels right or wrong in your body. I've always been a highly sensitive human and when the emotions and chaos of the outer world became too much to take on for my inner world, I learned how to dissociate and numb out.

This would serve me well as I pushed myself to be an A student and partake in every extracurricular in the handbook of how to be an overachiever. If I didn't have to feel my body, then I could dismiss any and all cues that I was hitting an edge and keep powering through.

I got really good at this, so when my back started to hurt with no apparent injury I was beyond confused and felt embarrassed that no doctors could find a root cause. I was 17 years old at the time and I couldn't get through a full day of classes without several high-dose narcotics. I had seen 17 different doctors who all kept pushing me off to the next and the number of pain medications I was on kept growing to the point where I would have needed a pain pump next, had I continued the path I was on.

Then one day while I was at my high school's homecoming parade, I went from feeling fine and watching floats go by to passing out on the ground and throwing up. I had accidentally overdosed on the pain pills. Even though it would still be years until I realized how disconnected from my body I was, that was a pivotal moment in knowing that pain medication was not the solution for me.

Resilience Redefined

I stopped using the narcotics and saw a rheumatologist who finally diagnosed me with fibromyalgia. My memory of his explanation of this common "catch-all" diagnosis goes something like this: "It's chronic widespread pain without a known cause; it could be all in your head." And the treatment? Antidepressants.

I was devastated. The pain had gotten so debilitating I had to quit the soccer team and was starting to be made fun of for the pain "ticks" I had developed. And now this doctor was basically confirming my fear that I had made all this up in my head? It was too much to digest, yet I lacked any other tools, resources, or confidence to do anything but fill the prescription and continue to numb my body (and now my emotions too).

Dissociation became my friend, and, in some ways, it actually did protect me. I wouldn't have known how to cope with everything in my life if I could feel the depth of emotions and pain truly present. But after four years of beer pong leagues, pulling all-nighters in the library, and eating highly processed foods, I was bloated nearly every day, I was constantly fatigued, and the pain was still there. So, when I walked out of that yoga class and back into my body I was overwhelmed, but in a "this is what I've been looking for" kind of way.

Deciding to Take Care of Myself

I started to feel again. It began with feeling my low back press against the floor, then my fingers touching my toes, and then my breathing corrected after years of reverse breathing—now, on each inhale my belly expanded instead of contracted. I felt myself slowly building back body awareness that had previously felt unmanageable. I was coming back home to myself (or at least my physical body) and yoga was the gateway that led me there.

I didn't just flirt with feeling my body again; I dove all the way in. I declined a high school biology teacher position in Chicago after college graduation and decided to become a yoga teacher. After a year of breathing this movement practice into my body every single day and teaching it to others full-time, I couldn't just touch my toes, I could feel every part of my body inside and out again. That's when I started to notice the signs my body had been giving me all along. My face was covered in cystic acne, my hands were raw from eczema, and all my joints were inflamed. It was time to seek deeper answers.

Back then I thought that maybe yoga was the cure to all my maladies, but really it was just what pulled back the veil. I moved to Chicago to work on my master's degree and finally found a holistic practitioner who saw me as a whole being instead of a segment of parts. I was diagnosed with anxiety, celiac disease, and hormone imbalance. I had also developed a staph infection in my nose that took several rounds of antibiotics to resolve. While the antibiotics were creating havoc in my gut microbiome, I was slowly working on changing my diet and adding supplements that would replenish my gut bacteria and bring down my inflammation.

Removing gluten from my diet was... a process. I had never even heard about gluten before being diagnosed with celiac disease. I thought not eating bread and pasta would pretty much do the trick. I was wrong. When my eczema was still persistent, my hands were still wrapped in bandages from how raw they were, and my stomach rash was biopsied for leukemia (which came back negative), I decided to actually do the research to understand all the hidden places gluten lives. And if you, dear reader, are also living a gluten-free life, you know that it's all sorts of places from your shampoo to lip balm to supplements to soy sauce, and of course our beloved baked goods.

Once I committed to the process, living a gluten-free life became second nature and I fully embraced being a gluten-free girlie. But interestingly, I still didn't associate this allergy as being an autoimmune disease. I did slowly watch my eczema dissolve, my feet shrank two sizes as my body released inflammation, and my digestion felt much better, but I still had lingering symptoms and my skin continued to be the alert system for when something was off. I was starting to lose pigment in my skin and my anxious feelings were starting to skyrocket. I would regularly pull over my car on the verge of a panic attack. These full-body episodes struck out of nowhere and they truly convinced me I was dying.

One night I came home to my apartment and had a particularly bad panic attack in the middle of my living room floor. I lay there feeling helpless and hopeless, wondering when these emotional storms would stop tormenting me. The next morning, I received a dozen phone calls from my family telling me my younger brother took his life that evening.

This came as a shock and the tidal wave of grief caused all the walls of perfection and emotional repression to collapse. I could no longer pretend that just being aware of my physical body was enough to fully heal; my emotions needed attention too. All of the efforts I had funneled into keeping my shit together suddenly evaporated. It just so happened that the insurmountable loss of my brother was the catalyst for feeling again. So, I let grief have its way with me. I was enraged, heartbroken, confused, and so, so sad. I let my grief overflow and invited in any and all emotions from other past life experiences to have their way with me too. It was exhausting... and beautiful.

Shortly after my brother passed, when I was in the pits of emotional exhaustion, I learned what an empath was. My mom shared this term with me and suddenly my whole life made more sense. An empath is someone who takes on another's feelings and energy as their own, like an emotional (and sometimes physical) sponge. This is why the world had always felt like too much and why I always felt so sensitive, especially to other people's emotions. I was ecstatic to have a word for my life experience and, more importantly, to know that I wasn't alone and that maybe the physical intensity I had experienced at age 17 wasn't actually all in my head.

I know now that being an empath doesn't automatically lead to chronic illness, but being an empath without any tools for emotional and nervous system regulation can certainly lead to feeling overwhelmed. A dysregulated nervous system has a laundry list of effects on your physical body like impaired digestion, increased heart rate, shallow breathing, and more. The long-term effects of nervous system imbalance paired with trauma and chronic stress created a perfect breeding ground for autoimmune disease in my body.

The Tools I Use to Thrive

Not long after this newfound knowledge, I was inspired to leave my career in sustainable food systems and start doing more of what I love on my own terms. It was during this time that I found the holistic healing lineup of functional medicine, energy healing, breathwork, Emotional Freedom Technique (EFT), somatic healing, and mindset work. Through functional lab testing, I discovered how much more was going on in my body than I ever realized (and why my daily and debilitating panic attacks weren't going away with happy thoughts and healthy food).

The results showed a myriad of factors that were contributing to feeling unwell, including heavy metal toxicity, high oxalates, parasites, hormone imbalance, bacterial infections like H. pylori and C. diff, candida, high inflammation, adrenal fatigue, liver stagnation, genetic mutations like MTHFR and COMT, mold illness, vitiligo, and chronic inflammatory response syndrome (CIRS). I distinctly remember the video call with my practitioner to go over all these results. He approached the discussion with such care, under what I presume was the assumption that this would be a lot to digest and overcome. I listened intently. Yes, it was a lot of information to digest, but the overarching message I heard from his voice was hope. You don't know what you don't know, and you can't heal what you aren't aware of. I felt like a veil had been lifted and information was flooding in. Information that I could do something with and start the long healing journey ahead of me.

Ever since I had started feeling my body and my emotions again, I knew intuitively that something was out of balance, not right, call it what you will... but with these results I could stop guessing what to do next and address each problem appropriately and holistically. Two years later my life was completely different. I had been through dozens of bottles of supplements, quite a few coffee enemas, and lots of nutrient-dense food all to feel alive again. And slowly (and let me tell you, it was a process) I started to get my energy back, my skin cleared up, my digestion was no longer painful, and best of all, I wasn't having panic attacks anymore. I changed nearly every product I was using on my body and in my home. I changed the way I ate. I changed the way I slept. I changed the way I spoke to myself in the mirror. I changed the way I managed stress. I changed my relationship dynamics. I changed the way I took care of my energy. And though it was definitely a hard path filled with detox symptoms and label scouring and exhaustion, it was more than worth it to remember who I was inside.

Admittedly, there were several years when I was so invested in feeling better that the quest for health seemed to take over my life. But when the fog lifted, I could start to see who I was underneath all the symptoms: someone who wanted to live a wild and beautiful life and feel well enough to experience the depth of emotions available to us as human beings. So, once I started to feel well, I made a vow to myself to never let the intuitive feeling that something was off in my body go unanswered again.

Becoming more intimately aware of the language of my intuition, especially as a sensitive empath, allowed me to navigate red flags as they popped up. How this played out was always different, but I was committed to listening. For example, a few years ago I was intuitively led to a documentary on the dental industry, which got me thinking about the six screws I had in my jaw from a lower mandible extension I had when I was 16 years old. The surgery was slightly botched, and I had had chronic jaw pain ever since. This intuitive hunch led me to get a cone beam scan with a holistic dentist and, sure enough, I had an infection on one of my back lower molars where a screw was poorly positioned. I ended up getting the tooth removed and was quite shocked to see a large portion of the melasma on my face disappear and my jaw pain decreased significantly.

Then, in 2020, I got pregnant. I recorded a short video of me in the bathroom calling my husband in to tell him I was pregnant amidst a global pandemic. We were thrilled (and slightly terrified). We told all our closest friends and family, but something felt off. I started to feel some pain that was hard to describe, but the clearest way I could put it was like a Lego was stuck inside me. I called the midwife's office and requested to be seen. They were confused why I was there so early on in my pregnancy, but after they ordered the blood work and did the ultrasound I requested, it was confirmed I had a tubal pregnancy (a type of ectopic pregnancy). While this was gut-wrenching and brought on new waves of grief, I was also fortunate that I listened to my intuition and was able to receive treatment before losing a fallopian tube, or, worse, having it burst.

Interestingly, I've been free of autoimmune flares for about four years, but as I prepared to contribute my story to this book, I was also juggling a lot in my personal life. I was the wedding planner for my sister's wedding. I'm a mom of two little girls aged two and five months now, we just sold a home and business, I'm operating my other business solo, and we had to say a really hard goodbye to my dog of 15 years just last week. It was during this time that my body started to communicate with me yet again. Eczema popped back up on my hands one knuckle at a time; by the third inflamed knuckle, I called my functional practitioner to run labs. There's a part of me from the past that would have felt like this was a failure or backtracking or like it was all my fault. But I've chosen to be much more tender with myself these days. Sometimes flares happen. For me, they are way more likely to happen when the parts of life that are out of control stack up. I accept the fact that my health may fluctuate as the circumstances of my environment change, but I don't panic because I know my body's resilience. I've felt this strength in my body again and again and again.

Knowing that I am a sensitive person means that I will always feel things more deeply. But sensitive souls can be like canaries in a coal mine. I know and trust my body will develop a headache nearly instantaneously when I enter a moldy home. I can smell an artificially scented plug-in immediately when we enter a vacation rental house. I can intuit my two-year-old's emotions and pick up on when she's about to hit her own sensory stimulation limit. All of these things help me protect myself and my family on an ongoing basis. Sensitivity has truly become one of my greatest strengths; it operates like an internal thermometer and intuitively guides me toward what is going to best support my health and tells me what to avoid.

Taking care of myself today looks like lots of bodywork and body awareness. I'm in constant communication with my body and its messages. My body craves sensory input that feels nourishing, like deep-pressure massages and warm salt baths. Whereas it sends little alarms when I'm about to hit sensory overload, like when the TV is too loud, or the environment is too crowded. I go to the chiropractor weekly to keep my fibromyalgia pain at bay. I eat nutrient-dense whole foods and stay hydrated. I get sun exposure and lots of time outside with my feet on the earth. I use yoga and meditation to ground myself and get curious. I use breathwork to open conversations with my higher self. I listen to my intuitive nudges and follow them. I utilize subconscious reprogramming methods like tapping and hypnosis to rewire old, unsupportive beliefs into ones that align with my desires. I give myself many outlets to be creative. I prioritize silliness and laughter through playing with my girls. I check in with my nervous system daily, even if that means acknowledging it's way out of whack. I forgive myself and I reparent my inner child. I keep learning. I order functional lab tests as needed. And I carry the belief that my body and being are resilient. They can overcome. They can heal. They can evolve. They can do hard things.

Mindset Work

I don't consider myself perfectly healed. I'm not sure such a thing exists. What I do know is that it's possible to live a life you love with an autoimmune disease. To thrive in the thorniest conditions and find yourself again. To remember what it feels like to be in your body and live with a passion, especially because you know what it feels like to be debilitatingly ill. The tools I mentioned above are not things I do every single day—that wouldn't be sustainable for me as a mom of a toddler and a baby—but they are the foundation of my well-being. I tap into each as the cycles of my body flow. Having this multidimensional toolbox allows me to live without the fear cloud that used to follow me around, threatening another panic attack, another infection or another outbreak. That fear cloud finally turned into a cleansing rain when I committed to loving myself. That commitment built self-trust. It let me know that my body was trustworthy.

I believe healing inevitably leads you to your life's purpose. It has certainly helped me create a body of work that will be my legacy and one that I am proud of. To those of you still in the trenches, I see you. Keep following your intuitive nudges. Let our stories of resilience breathe hope into your body.

7
Healthier Because of Multiple Sclerosis

Sarah Wilson

Resilience is when you take circumstances that come your way and you are able to learn and put into action tools that help you come out stronger. In my case, I am healthier and more knowledgeable about myself, and my health and I thank the diagnosis of MS for that.

I would like to dedicate my chapter to my husband Dwayne. My diagnosis was completely unexpected and the ways in which you stepped up to support me have been a true blessing. You have been my rock and some days you believe in me more than I do myself. Thank you for the love and sense of safety you bring to my life every day.

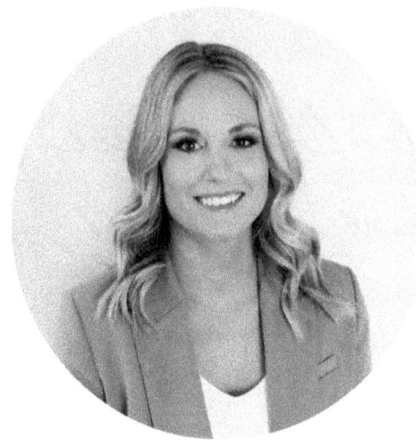

SARAH WILSON

Sarah Wilson lives in Alberta, is a wife to her high school sweetheart Dwayne, mom to two boys Nick & Andrew and has supported families who have children with autism for 18 years. After being diagnosed with MS in 2008, she's gone from completely lost in denial to fear and now out the other side to thriving. She knows that she is healthier because of MS. Sarah has a passion for sharing with others how she turned her path around and enjoys speaking to those newly diagnosed. When she's not working or spending time with her boys she loves working out, spending time outside, and being in the Rocky Mountains.

Diagnosis Story

Let's go back to June 2008, when you would find me at the age of 26 sitting in the Edmonton International Airport with my favorite Lululemon outfit, Starbucks, an Emily Giffin book, and all the excitement of going to Ottawa to see my younger sister graduate from university. All was fine—and in an instant, I noticed my right eye hurt when I moved it left or right. I thought I was just getting a headache and ignored the pain during the flight. By the time I landed the pain was stronger. I carried on with my family that evening, but it was getting harder to not let the pain and discomfort affect me.

The following day, we all got in the car to drive five hours to Guelph, where the graduation was. As we were driving, I couldn't help but notice that the signs along the highways were clear for my left eye, but blurry for my right eye, to the point that I could not read them. I remember spending most of the drive covering my left eye just to keep confirming that I, in fact, could hardly see out my right, maybe wishing for it to get better. Fast forward to when it was time for me to fly back to Edmonton a couple of days later, and I was completely blind in my right eye. For me, things did not go black but instead just pure white. At this point, I was still thinking something simple had happened, some sort of infection, maybe?

When I landed, I went right to an optometrist. For some reason, my saying, "I am blind in my right eye" prompted her to do the peripheral vision test where you push a button every time you see the little black line appear. She tested my right eye first and after a few minutes of me not pushing the button even once, she realized how severe this was. She told me that she was referring me to an ophthalmologist as they deal with more severe cases. The next day I got the call that I had an appointment at the eye clinic at the local hospital. Again, I explained I was blind in the right eye, but they wanted to complete a vision test, just to be sure. I sat in the chair and the tech asked me to read the letters on the top line. Well, I could not even see the room I was in, let alone the letters. Then, the tech stood up at the door and said, "Can you see my face?" and I said, "No, I see nothing." Next, I was called in to finally see the ophthalmologist, and he said, "You will be referred to see a neurologist next. You have optic neuritis, which is the first sign of multiple sclerosis."

To this day, I get asked what that moment was like, hearing that I may have MS, and my response is always, "I felt nothing; I did not really hear the words or let that sink in." From June to October, while I waited to see the neurologist, I went on with my regular life. My eye slowly healed, and my vision returned to normal after six weeks.

In October 2008, I had my first neurologist appointment and my first MRI, where I realized just how claustrophobic I am. On November 14, 2008, I experienced hearing, "You have multiple sclerosis" and "If you wanted to have children, the sooner the better, as pregnancy is good for MS and best to do before you start the medication." I left that office with my husband, Dwayne, and my mom as if we were leaving the mall. I had no response, no feelings, no fear, and no acceptance of the diagnosis I had just received.

The next three years were dedicated to being pregnant and having my two amazing sons, Nick and Andrew. I do not think I thought of my diagnosis at all unless I had an appointment or someone else brought it up. I left everything to do with MS back in my neurologist's office on the day of diagnosis.

After I came out of the newborn fog for both boys, which included a rough go of postpartum depression with my first, I started to not feel well. This is when MS started to impact my, and therefore my family's, life. I did not have another MS flare, but I just did not feel well. The year 2012, let's say, is when I felt like a truly sick person and every day I was reminded of my diagnosis. I was so tired, had severe vertigo, tingles, vibrations in my legs and feet, and just was not myself. My husband would have to take days off work so he could be with the kids while I rested. You can imagine what that did to our finances, and we are still recovering today.

For the next four years, I just existed and pushed through each day and was in bed on the days I could not push anymore. When my husband and I reflect we cannot believe how much time I spent laying on the couch. I still did not talk about MS or how it was making me feel with anyone outside of Dwayne, as the more people acknowledged my current state, the more real it was. I was blessed to not have any further "attacks" but rather symptoms of the disease and I was not on any disease-modifying treatments. I avoided that conversation like the plague until February 2016 when, after an MRI, it was finally my reality. I met with the nurse for a medication teaching session where they brought out all the pamphlets and showed me how each medication would work, where I would inject myself, how often, and the reality of what my body would look like after years of these injections, and which ones were best based on the side effects. An alarm went off inside me during this appointment as I was told that most people would take their meds on a Friday so if they felt sick, they could feel sick on the weekend and not have it impact their work. My mind started to spin, as I am so very sensitive to all medication and what most people feel for 2–4 hours, I feel for 8–12. My thoughts immediately went to wondering, *how am I going to lose my weekends with my family and possibly days of work following the injection, all to feel better, maybe? Was this a better quality of life?*

Deciding to Take Care of Myself

I remember like it was yesterday what it was like leaving that nurse's office, with all the pamphlets and a storybook on MS for my kids, thinking, could there be more that I could learn and do for my body, for my health?

Only a few days later, as if it was fate, I started to see different accounts and information on social media about living well with MS by changing my diet and lifestyle. Living well with MS, I still remember thinking. I had never heard those words in the same phrase.

This immediately intrigued me, and so I did some research and read some books including Healing Multiple Sclerosis by Ann Boroch, The Wahls Protocol by Terry Wahls, M.D., and The Autoimmune Paleo Cookbook by Mickey Trescott. I also sought out people who could answer my questions.

I found the program that kick-started my healing journey. I still say to this day that this was the program that truly changed my journey with living with MS. It was the online 90-day program called Live Disease Free (https://livediseasefree.com/) being offered by Pam Bartha. With the support of my family, I registered and started my journey with her program. March 1, 2016, was day one of my new life and the first steps to living well with MS! It was during this program and the work I got to complete that some of the puzzle pieces came together in terms of the "why" behind my being diagnosed. As a child I suffered from ear infections and from childhood until early adulthood I had yearly strep throat infections, which meant many rounds of antibiotics. Also, when I was a teenager, I suffered from acne, and I was on Accutane to help relieve the physical and therefore emotional effects of acne and being a young woman. Reflecting and learning of the connections between all this and overall health was again the beginning of me piecing together how MS manifested in my body but, this was only the beginning and only some of the story.

The Tools I Use to Thrive

The following is what I have focused on and what my journey has looked like, in order, over the past seven years. The history of my wellness journey is a mix of the Live Disease Free program and other work I have done to achieve optimal health with MS.

Nutrition

The first step was diet, and I went all in instead of one thing at a time. Caffeine, alcohol, sugar, dairy, gluten, legumes, and grains of all kinds were eliminated! I still remember the awful three-day withdrawal headache, but I pushed through knowing this was it! The program came with a strict guide of what to eliminate and add and helpful recipes to try. A few years later I came across MS Hope and The Best Bet Diet, and this diet and cookbook put a name to the way I was eating! Sarah with a lunch bag was the new norm. No matter where we were going or who we were with, I was confident to bring my own food and drink so that I always had an option and never let myself be hungry. The lesson here is, do not be shy and do what you need to stay on track! This was a great start to my journey, but it was only the beginning.

Supplements

While I adjusted my eating habits and got used to my new meals (vegetables for breakfast was a hard pill to swallow at first) and all the new food prep needed, the next step was supplements and protocols for further healing. After about two weeks of eating clean and getting into my new groove with food, with the help of the program and a new naturopathic doctor, I explored cleanses and protocols that could be done to further my experience of health with MS. Finding a naturopathic doctor that would partner with me on my journey and help guide me along further was so key to success. This practitioner ordered further bloodwork and testing in order to guide me on what more my body needed in order to stay balanced and healthy. Taking the right kind and amounts of supplements and using some simple protocols helped my body turn another corner to wellness. This journey to optimal health was an investment for my family, as going off the typical health road came with a cost, though it's one we will never regret. The biggest lesson here is to know that supplements are never a cure, always take what your body needs based on bloodwork and/or as recommended by your healthcare provider and remember this is not where your health journey will end.

Walking Away from Western Medicine

By the time my birthday came around in May—two months after I'd started the Live Disease Free program—I knew I was feeling different, but this was also when others were starting to notice the shift as well. I was down a significant amount of weight, and I was no longer lying on the couch after work and all weekend due to fatigue. My symptoms were hardly noticeable if at all and I was living and loving life again! I was so passionate about this new and beautiful way of living that it became who I was, and I shared it with anyone who wanted to listen.

From May 2016 to August 2017, I continued with my new way of eating, using supplements and doing cleanses based on my bloodwork and recommendations from my health practitioner and the Live Disease Free program. I felt better and better as each week went on and I can honestly say I looked better and healthier than I did before diagnosis. In August 2017 I was scheduled for a follow-up MRI and appointment with my neurologist, and I could not wait!

I remember so clearly walking into that office and being called to the back. For once I had no fear, just excitement to show them the changes in me and how well I was living my life. The first stop was to get weighed, and

I was down 35 pounds, which made an alarm on the machine go off—I guess that much of a weight difference was a concern. Next, into the room, I went to meet with my doctor, who shared that I had no active lesions (no active disease) and no new lesions when compared to my previous MRI. This was huge and only solidified that what I had been doing was working! She commented and recognized how well I looked and how well I was obviously doing. I shared everything I'd been doing with such passion and authenticity, hoping that she might share it with other patients who could use this information. Unfortunately, her response was less than ideal, and the end result of the appointment was her saying, and I quote, "It looks like you have chosen your path with how to deal with having MS, but I am trained in Western medicine, and I cannot let myself believe that what you are doing will have long-standing effects. We no longer need to have our yearly follow-ups, but I will always be your neurologist if you need one."

I left that office standing so tall and feeling so proud of who I was, what I had done for my health, and how I tried to share information with her that she could pass on to other patients. Choosing whether to take medication is a personal choice and one that should never be judged, but changing your lifestyle and becoming your own advocate could help anyone. After 15 years with MS, she and I should have another conversation, because this is definitely what I consider a long-standing success!

Movement

I was always active and loved to run and lift weights, but I never knew exercise could be a part of my plan for living healthy with MS. Once I knew this, my entire relationship and respect for movement changed. Over the years, I have built myself a strong foundation of practices that I implement without fail: yoga (1–2x a week), weights (4x a week), and cardio (2x a week, plus daily walks). I am so thankful for my body and the ability to move like I do, and I never take this for granted.

Awareness of Toxic Load

Throughout my journey, I would say within the last 4 years specifically, is when I came to understand that not only does what we put in our body via food and drink impact our health, it is equally important to review what we are using on our bodies and in our homes! I switched to natural cleaning products, laundry detergent, creams I use on my body and diffusing dōTERRA oils vs using candles. When reviewing what you are using for your body care and in your home, the process can be overwhelming and an investment! Go slow and start with one area at a time to help you be successful. Remember, our toxic load impacts our overall health and is an important piece to address for overall wellness.

Another addition to my and my family's overall shift away from toxicity has been homeopathy! Our medicine cabinet went from Tylenol, Advil and cough syrup to a variety of homeopathy remedies and books to educate what remedy we take for what acute condition. When you put the effort in and learn how to look after your family's health, there is such a sense of power!

Sleep

I have worked hard to get where I am with sleep. My nighttime routine is strong, and I rarely deviate from it. I notice how my body does not feel its best if I do not stay on routine and schedule. My evenings consist of nightly Epsom salt baths, dimmed lights, relaxing music, castor oil packs, and a consistent bedtime to ensure I get eight hours of sleep. If you do not find what works for you to get good quality sleep, you will continue to struggle because sleep is part of the foundation for good health just like nutrition.

Boundaries

Something that has only recently started to be comfortable for me but is so important to my healing is setting boundaries for myself. I was always a "yes" girl growing up and into adulthood. Lately, I have come to feel the positive effects of doing what serves me and not only serving others. I now set strong boundaries with how I spend my time and I do not participate in anything that does not feel good to me or that I know will interrupt my routines. I also feel it is important to get comfortable with advocating for yourself within your career. Finding a workplace that allows employees to look after their health is important for both productivity at work and our wellbeing. I have been so fortunate to work at an organization that implements sick days, work from home options and a flexible schedule. I truly believe that this has allowed me to work and grow in my career while working on my healing journey without having to choose one or the other, and for that I am grateful.

Mindset Work

I have come to learn from experience that your mindset around your health and/or disease is more important than anything else. You can be doing all the things, but if at your core you do not believe that you can live well with your diagnosis, you will always be working against yourself.

In 2021, I was having a hard time with the pandemic and all the isolation that came with it. My mindset around my health came to a crashing moment of complete fear even without changes and I knew I needed to do some work in this area. I continued with all my daily practices, but I also added a psychologist to my team. With her help, I came to recognize that although I was living very well with this disease and had become confident and more knowledgeable about my diagnosis and what I implement to live well, there was deeper work to be done. I needed to go back 15 years, to the time of diagnosis. I was able to bring myself back to that first neurologist appointment when I was diagnosed and face my diagnosis that day. I let myself acknowledge what this diagnosis felt like at that moment. By the time we completed the bulk of our work together around this, I felt free. I worked through how I felt about the diagnosis on day one and then how I feel about the diagnosis today. I often say that having MS is a gift because it makes me take care of myself better than I was before or would be without it! I am a healthier version of myself, even with MS.

My mindset has gone through a rollercoaster from denial to complete fear and now out the other side where I accept and take ownership of this disease and how I can support my body today and always.

I have worked really hard to have the mindset of knowing I will live well with MS, that I am safe, and that

I give my body all the support it needs to live in optimal health. Mindset tools I have used and still use today include boundaries, journaling, meditation, mirror work, affirmations, and therapy when needed. I wish I could give more concrete tools, but it really comes down to internal thoughts around this diagnosis.

My current library of daily practices brings me such peace and keeps me from being thrown into fear and anxiety. The next steps include continued work with my naturopath and those that specialize in root causes, as there is always more to learn about my body and where imbalances remain.

To close out my story, I have watched myself go through different versions of Sarah and where I have landed is so beautiful. It makes me smile to know that MS is not devastating nor the end of me as it has brought so much good to my life! I have had the opportunity to be interviewed on my journey with MS and participate in MS wellness groups on social media. I have been available to meet, text, email, or call anyone newly diagnosed, as well as their relatives, who needed someone to chat with. I am so passionate about how I live my life and sharing in any way I can with others. MS is not something I would say I want; however, so many beautiful people, opportunities, and knowledge about my long-term health came into my life because of this diagnosis. When I share that I have MS, my most disliked response is the head-tilt and "I'm sorry" comment. I do not need sympathy; I need curiosity and the opportunity to share my story and how for 15 years I have lived so well with MS. I will continue being a student, someone who empowers others, a collaborator, and a researcher for my overall well-being and if and when I need to pivot my approach, I will be open to what comes next. I have MS but I am not MS. I am an MS Thriver. To me, that means staying true to myself, first and foremost, while being my own advocate, researcher, and guiding light to optimal health. Accepting me as me and each day as it comes with a positive mindset.

www.ingramcontent.com/pod-product-compliance
Lightning Source LLC
Chambersburg PA
CBHW071715020426
42333CB00017B/2274